Advanced and Specialist Nursing Practice

Advanced and Specialist Nursing Practice

Edited by

George Castledine and Paula McGee

**Blackwell
Science**

© 1998 by
Blackwell Science Ltd
Editorial Offices:
Osney Mead, Oxford OX2 0EL
25 John Street, London WC1N 2BL
23 Ainslie Place, Edinburgh EH3 6AJ
350 Main Street, Malden
  MA 02148 5018, USA
54 University Street, Carlton
  Victoria 3053, Australia
10, rue Casimir Delavigne
  75006 Paris, France

Other Editorial Offices:

Blackwell Wissenschafts-Verlag GmbH
Kurfürstendamm 57
10707 Berlin, Germany

Blackwell Science KK
MG Kodenmacho Building
7-10 Kodenmacho Nihombashi
Chuo-ku, Tokyo 104, Japan

The right of the Author to be identified as the
Author of this Work has been asserted in
accordance with the Copyright, Designs and
Patents Act 1988.

First published 1998

Set in 10/12.5 pt Palatino
by DP Photosetting, Aylesbury, Bucks
Printed and bound in Great Britain by
The University Press, Cambridge

The Blackwell Science logo is a
trade mark of Blackwell Science Ltd,
registered at the United Kingdom
Trade Marks Registry

DISTRIBUTORS

Marston Book Services Ltd
PO Box 269
Abingdon
Oxon OX14 4YN
(*Orders:* Tel: 01235 465500
        Fax: 01235 465555)

USA
Blackwell Science, Inc.
Commerce Place
350 Main Street
Malden, MA 02148 5018
(*Orders:* Tel: 800 759 6102
        781 388 8250
        Fax: 781 388 8255)

Canada
Login Brothers Book Company
324 Saulteaux Crescent
Winnipeg, Manitoba R3J 3T2
(*Orders:* Tel: 204 837 2987
        Fax: 204 837 3116)

Australia
Blackwell Science Pty Ltd
54 University Street
Carlton, Victoria 3053
(*Orders:* Tel: 03 9347 0300
        Fax: 03 9347 5001)

A catalogue record for this title
is available from the British Library

ISBN 0-632-04248-6

Library of Congress
Cataloging-in-Publication Data
Advanced and specialist nursing practice/
  edited by George Castledine, Paula McGee.
    p. cm.
  Includes bibliographical references and
index.
  ISBN 0-632-04248-6
  1. Nursing specialties—Great Britain.
  2. Nursing specialties—United States.
  I. Castledine, George. II. McGee, Paula.
  [DNLM 1. Specialties, Nursing—Great
Britain. 2. Specialties, Nursing–
United States. WY 101 A243 1998]
RT89.A38 1998
  610.73′6′0941–dc21
  DNLM/DLC
  for Library of Congress   98-25008
                                              CIP

For further information on
Blackwell Science, visit our website:
www.blackwell-science.com

To Ruth Martin and all those like her who influenced our early thinking.
To all specialist and advanced nurses past and present.

Contents

Preface

The publication of standards for post-registration education and practice (UKCC, 1994) attempted, for the first time, to provide a comprehensive definition of specialist nursing. In doing so, the United Kingdom Central Council (UKCC) was trying to clarify a level of practice which had, until then, developed in a rather piecemeal fashion. The object was to produce a definition and standards in education which could be used as a yardstick by nurses for determining whether or not they were truly specialist practitioners. At the same time, the UKCC introduced the concept of advanced practice, recognizing that some nurses might not wish to become specialists but were nevertheless capable of making significant contributions to nursing. These individuals were seen as functioning on the frontiers of the profession, advancing practice and exploring the interface with other professionals.

This book aims to explore the concepts of specialist and advanced practice as they are developing in the UK. This exploration incorporates the experiences of nurses working as specialist and advanced practitioners. It also includes perspectives from academics in the UK and the USA where the concepts of specialist and advanced practice are well established, although their expression is not the same. These contributions are a unique feature of the book in that this is the first time that ideas about specialist and advanced practice from the two countries have been addressed side by side in this way.

The book is intended primarily for those who are, or who are studying to become, specialist or advanced practitioners. However, it is anticipated that managers and other senior personnel who have responsibilities for such posts will also find it useful. We also hope that nurses at the beginning of their careers will find it helpful in gaining an understanding of the current issues in specialist and advanced practice and in looking to their own futures.

In Chapters 1 and 2, George Castledine explains the historical development of specialist and advanced practice in the UK in order to contextualize the publication of the UKCC's standards. This is the first time that such a comprehensive account has been available and it has the additional advantage of insight from a nurse who has participated in this development. The chapter will be extremely helpful to students, tutors and practitioners as it introduces the reader to the various, sometimes contradictory, developments which culminated in the Council's standards. Alongside specialist and advanced roles, there have been experiments with other possibilities, such as the nurse practitioner and the physician's assistant roles. The physician's assistant role in particular is not well understood in the UK and this chapter clarifies both these roles.

Chapters 1 and 2 are balanced by an account of the development of specialist and advanced practice in the United States. Ann Hamric's work on the clinical nurse specialist is well known (Hamric and Spross, 1989) and underpins Part 2 of this book in which examples of current British specialist roles are examined. Chapter 3 culminates in the presentation of her latest work. This proposes that advanced practitioners, irrespective of their job titles, should be able to master certain specified competencies. In doing so, the current confusion between clinical nurse specialists, nurse practitioners, advanced practice nurses and many other titles might be eliminated. These ideas are applied in Part 3 of this book in which five British advanced practice roles are discussed.

As nursing practice continues to develop, questions naturally arise about the legal dimensions of their work. This is particularly likely to occur when individuals are challenging the boundaries of existing practice and seeking to adopt new roles. In Chapter 4, John Tingle draws attention to some of the potential consequences which may arise. Each nurse must be aware of his/her limitations in terms of knowledge and skill but even highly competent practitioners can find themselves in difficulties. Strategies such as good record keeping and effective communication systems are an essential part of good practice at every level of nursing, but they are particularly important when the individual steps outside what is generally considered to be accepted nursing work. Allied to this is the need for research not only to extend and develop nursing knowledge but also to demonstrate the effectiveness of changes in practice. Chapter 5 outlines the first survey of the employment of specialist and advanced practitioners by NHS trusts in England and discusses ideas for future research.

Chapter 6 covers a specific area of nursing skill for both specialist and advanced practitioners. Advanced health assessment skills are essential for nurses seeking to extend and develop their practice. Susan Cohen and her colleagues practise both in the clinical arena and in the educational setting. They are therefore ideally placed to link theory to practice in demonstrating the nature and level of physical assessment skills. This is achieved through the presentation of three case studies of patients with a range of complex problems. These illustrate the knowledge base required by the nurse as well as the level of skill needed to apply it. Competency is therefore a key issue. Sue Lillyman's chapter (Chapter 7) presents an analysis of this concept and the issues which might lie ahead if British nurses choose to use it as a basis for defining specialist and advanced nursing practice.

In Parts 2 and 3, the experiences of specialist and advanced practitioners are presented and discussed. Individual practitioners have contributed descriptions of certain aspects of their work and the ideas of Hamric (1996) and Benner *et al.* (1996) are used to inform the discussion. Part 2 addresses specialist practice by examining the role of five nurses, including an HIV/AIDS nurse, a nutrition nurse specialist and a cultural liaison officer. This part of the book spans hospital and community work but also incorporates perspectives from the independent health care sector. This is a unique feature of the book which, to the best of our knowledge, has not been covered elsewhere in any other British publication. Each nurse outlines two or three aspects of his/her role. This is not intended as a comprehensive account but as a means of providing examples of the work undertaken. These examples are then compared and contrasted in order to identify differences and similarities between specialist nurses in very diverse fields.

Part 3 takes the same approach to advanced practice. Five advanced practitioners present accounts of some aspects of their work. These practitioners represent the fields of mental health, cardiology, accident and emergency, care of older people and learning disabilities nursing. The accounts presented provide examples of the work these nurses undertake and allow similarities and differences to be identified across disciplinary boundaries.

In the final part of this book, we present our vision of the future for specialist and advanced practice in Britain. This spans a wide range of issues which includes professional regulation and the possible impact of changes in government policy. Overall it is a vision which we think will take nursing into the twenty-first century.

George Castledine
Paula McGee

References

Benner, P., Tanner, C. and Chesla, C. (1996) *Expertise in Nursing Practice. Caring, clinical judgement and ethics.* Springer-Verlag, New York.

Hamric, A.B. (1996) A definition of advanced nursing practice. In: *Advanced Nursing Practice: an Integrative Approach* (eds A.B. Hamric, J.A. Spross & C.M. Hanson). W.B. Saunders, Philadelphia.

Hamric, A. and Spross, J. (1989) *The Clinical Nurse Specialist in Theory and Practice*, 2nd edn. W.B. Saunders, Philadelphia.

United Kingdom Central Council for Nursing Midwifery and Health Visiting (1994) *The Future of Professional Practice – the Council's Standards for Education and Practice Following Registration.* UKCC, London.

Acknowledgements

This book could not have been written without the help of many friends, colleagues and students who have given up their time to help us, listen to our ideas and give us their honest opinions. Their advice has enabled us to develop our thinking and create this book.

List of Contributors

Elizabeth Alsbury, RN, Dip. Psych., has been a lecturer practitioner in the independent health care sector for two years. She has developed a pre-admission clinic and a pain control team within the hospital in which she is based. Her additional responsibilities include facilitating the educational needs of staff, implementing clinical supervision and assisting in the introduction of care pathways and nursing audit. She participates in the provision of education for the whole company through the Advancing Practice Research Group.

Helen Arrowsmith, RN, DPSN, is a clinical nurse specialist at Birmingham and Solihull NHS Trust (Teaching) whose primary role is to enhance the care of patients requiring nutritional support in hospital and the community. She has recently served as secretary to the national nurses nutrition group for two years.

Patricia Polgar Bailey, MSN, CFNP, is a programme instructor in Nursing at Yale University and a nurse practitioner in the Yale New Haven Hospital Primary Care Centre, New Haven, Connecticut, USA. She is a certified family nurse practitioner.

Clarice Begemann, MSN, MPPM, CFNP, is a programme instructor in Nursing at Yale University and a nurse practitioner at the Fair Haven Community Health Center, New Haven, Connecticut, USA. She is a certified family nurse practitioner.

George Castledine, MSc, BA (Hons), Dip. Soc. Std. PGCE, RN, RNT, FRCN, is Professor of Nursing and Community Health and Assistant Dean in the Faculty of Health and Community Care at the University of Central England. He was Vice President of the United Kingdom Central Council for Nurses, Midwives and Health Visitors from 1993–8. He has conducted research into specialist and advanced nursing in the UK. He is a founding member of the Specialist and Advanced Practice Nurses Association and is President of the Infection Control Nurses Association.

Susan Cohen, DSN, CFNP, is an Associate Professor and Director of Adult and Faculty and Family Nurse Practitioner Program, Yale University, New Haven, Connecticut, USA. She is a certified family nurse practitioner and a researcher in the area of mid-life women's health.

Monica David, RN, is the Cultural Liaison Officer at Dudley Health Authority. Her remit is to identify the health care needs of black and minority ethnic people in Dudley and promote the targeting of services to meet their needs. She previously worked in occupational health in the private sector for many years and also spent two years working as a practice nurse.

Patricia Elliott, MSc, BEd, Cert. Ed., RN, ONC, DN (Lond.), RCNT, MICHT, is currently employed as an advanced nursing practitioner in the Worcestershire Community NHS Healthcare Trust. Her role encompasses practice developments within the field of rehabilitation and care of older people, particularly within the community hospital setting. In addition to clinical practice, she has been responsible for the development of continuing education for nurses within the trust. As a qualified aromatherapist she has also integrated this skill into her practice and has developed an aromatherapy foundation course for carers.

Jenny La Fontaine, MA, RMN, DPSN, Cert. Ed., is currently team manager for two community mental health teams and a day hospital for older people who experience mental health difficulties. She is based in the Northern Birmingham Mental Health Trust but is also employed as a visiting lecturer at the University of Central England as well as providing freelance consultancy and training. She has a particular interest in developing the role of the nurse in working with older people, elder abuse and with families and caregivers.

Kate Gee, RN, BA (Hons), MSc, is the clinical nurse specialist/senior nurse for the Cardiac Directorate at the University Hospital Birmingham NHS Trust. Throughout her professional career she has had a keen interest in cardiology, with the primary focus on raising the profile of the specialist practice of cardiac nurses. She has researched the rehabilitation of cardiac patients who experience a second myocardial infarction. Her work includes ECG interpretation and its relevance to care, competency development, evidence-based nursing and developing advanced assessment skills for nurses providing thrombolysis in admission areas.

Ann Hamric, RN, PhD, is Associate Professor for the graduate nursing programme at the Louisiana State University Medical Center School of Nursing in New Orleans, USA. She is also the senior editor for *Advanced Nursing Practice: an Integrative Approach*, published by W.B. Saunders in Philadelphia.

Sue Lillyman, MA, BSc (Nursing), RN, RM, DPSN, PGCE, is Faculty Head of Quality Assurance at the University of Central England in Birmingham. She has been a nurse for over twenty years and has a wide range of clinical experience which includes acute and rehabilitation care settings. During the last eight years she has taught on diploma, degree and postgraduate nursing and multidisciplinary courses.

Paula McGee, MA, BA, PGCE, RN, RNT, is Nursing Research Fellow in the Faculty of Health and Community Care at the University of Central England in Birmingham. She has undertaken research into specialist and advanced practice, has published a number of articles relating to this and teaches topics related to these fields.

Kate Moffett, MSN, CFNP, is a programme instructor in Nursing at Yale University and Nurse Practitioner at the Yale New Haven Hospital Primary Care Center, New Haven, Connecticut, USA. She is a certified family practitioner.

Patricia Overton-Brown, MHS, BSc (Hons), DPNS, RN, is a joint appointee as advanced nurse practitioner/lecturer practitioner at Birmingham Heartlands and Solihull NHS Trust (Teaching) and the University of Central England. Her field of practice is accident and emergency nursing and she has a keen interest in the role of the emergency nurse practitioner and advanced trauma care nursing.

John Quirk, RGN, BSc, is the clinical nurse specialist in HIV/AIDS and sexual health for Bournewood Community Mental Health NHS Trust, Chertsey, Surrey. He served as chair of the HIV nursing society at the Royal College of Nursing and as chair of the South Thames HIV/AIDS clinical nurse specialist group 1995–7. In 1998 he was awarded a Florence Nightingale Foundation Travel Scholarship to undertake a study tour of Uganda to examine HIV/AIDS care provision, prevention and education programmes.

Fiona Rich, RNMH, MSc (Advanced nursing practice), BSc (Hons), DPSN, Cert. Ed. (HE), is senior lecturer in learning disabilities nursing studies at the University of Central England. She has undertaken research into the role of specialist and advanced nurses in learning disability nursing.

John Tingle, BA Law (Hons), Cert. Ed., MEd, Barrister, is Reader in Health Law and Director of the Centre for Health Law, Nottingham Law School, Nottingham Trent University. He has published numerous articles in the nursing press on the legal aspects of nursing and is co-editor with Alan Cribb of *Nursing Law and Ethics* (1995), Blackwell Science, Oxford. He is also editor of the UK's first journal on clinical risk management and the law, *Health Care Risk Report*. He speaks regularly on health issues to nurses and doctors in the UK and abroad.

Julie Worth, RGN, RMN, BSc, Dip. N., joined Nuffield Hospitals, a company providing independent health care, in 1993. In 1995 she became a lecturer practitioner attached to the company's nurse education centre and undertook research into the implementation of clinical supervision in an independent hospital. She was appointed a hospital matron in 1996 and sees her work as focused on the drive for excellence in the independent sector.

Part 1
Current Issues

Chapter 1
Clinical Specialists in Nursing in the UK: The Early Years

George Castledine

Introduction

In the United Kingdom the Nurses Registration Act 1919 identified four major specialties: sick children, mental nursing, care of the mentally handicapped and fever nursing. The fever part of the Register was discontinued in 1967 because of changes in sickness patterns. Changes and advances in medical science, however, are not the only reasons for the recognition and development of specialization and further training in nursing, as Weller (1971) pointed out:

'... the education of the 1980s for the paediatric nurse should include knowledge and understanding of sociological trends and their effect upon child care, greater emphasis on child development both physically and psychologically, within the community.'

If specialization infers a narrowing of the range of work to be done, and an increase in depth of knowledge and skill, then we must take the setting up of the first training school in nursing after the Crimean War by Florence Nightingale as the starting point for specialization and identification of clinical nursing in the United Kingdom. Prior to this, nursing was very much in the hands of drunken females of ill repute and poor morals (Maggs, 1978). It was considered something which anybody could do, some better than most depending on their inclination and common sense. Later, however, with the introduction of training schemes and the battles for registration, the care of patients changed from the hands of working class married women, who tended to stay for long periods on one ward, to younger men and women of varied class who tended to move from one ward to another because of their training needs.

It is important, however, to distinguish between 'specialization of nursing', for this is what the introduction of training and registration accomplished, to that of 'specialization in nursing', which is something slightly different. 'Specialization of nursing' is determined by outside events and influences in medicine and society; whereas 'specialization in nursing' is intrinsic and is determined by nurses for the good of the patient. Both forms of specialization are interrelated and together determine the boundaries of the profession. Early specialization of nursing helped to raise the status and establishment of nursing as a profession; the chief motivating force towards this was, as Brian Abel-Smith (1960) called them, 'the professionally conscious lady nurses'.

It was Florence Nightingale, however, who first identified the central tasks in patient care, which were the domain of the nurse. Specialty was restricted to a particular facility or disease such as tuberculosis hospital, fever nursing or psychiatric care, and if a particular nurse was good at her job or performed very skilfully, little recognition was given except an invitation for a repeat performance or the status of being placed on a physician's list of expert nurses (Smoyak, 1976). Due to the lack of formal courses and an absence of research, it is very difficult to say if these early nurse experts were exceptionally good generalists or performed specific skills in depth.

It would seem, however, from examining nurse training syllabuses and noting the shortages of post-registration courses in clinical nursing, that up until the late 1960s nurse education in the UK was geared towards preparing and sustaining nurse generalists who tended to fit the saying 'jacks of all trades, masters of none'. Whyte (1977), reviewing some important events and developments in the hospital nursing service over the previous 25 years, felt that:

'the strangest influence on the pattern of nursing has been the changing attitude of society towards women. Their demand for independence, the pressure of economic factors, the changing patterns of marriage and child bearing, have all meant that women are now able to combine marriage with a career.'

In continuing her review of nursing, Whyte (1977) claimed that the profession has always consisted of two types of nurse:

'the Marthas who work with the patients, and the Marys who control and advise. The greatest change has been seen in the proportion of Mary's to Martha's, and this has been brought about by far reaching changes which have affected the whole structure of the Health Service. What might be termed "the management era of nursing" was ushered in by the Salmon and Mayston Reports.'

Austin (1977) criticized the Salmon Report (Mott, 1966) as 'the male nurses' charter' because it emphasized and approved male values, masculine knowledge and abilities, and the subordination of women to male bosses. Whatever the pros and cons of the Salmon Report, one crucial factor with regard to the development of specialization in nursing was that it diverted attention away from the clinical content of the nurse's role towards a more management-orientated approach.

There is no doubt that something has been happening in the relationship between nursing theory and practice, and perhaps because of this 'gulf' (Bendall, 1976, 1977), confusion arose as to which way clinical practice should develop. Also, there was little advice and guidance as to how deeply the clinical nurse should study nursing or medical knowledge. This anomaly led to some nurses developing their role around a medical model instead of a nursing one. It is interesting to note that the first movements in specialization in nursing took place not along clinical lines but along what are called 'functional specialties' such as administration, teaching and planning (Kohnke, 1978).

Referring to the 1940s and 1950s, Smoyak (1976) pointed out that most of the trained nurses' educational teaching curriculum 'focused on administration, teaching or supervision; clinical expertise was given lip service as a necessary component but was not reflected in course offerings'. The reason why this happened could have been because nurses were at one time seen as non-professionals, unable to assume self-direction and self-management, and therefore needing to be watched (Smoyak, 1976). This could account for the fact that of all the major organizational changes in nursing in the UK over recent years, the management structure designed by the Salmon Committee (Mott, 1966) was the most significant. In other countries such as the USA, the development of clinical specialization has been, in more recent times, linked with university education.

It appears that ideas were being put into practice in the late 1940s with regard to a clinical specialist educated at the master's level. The National League for Nursing in 1952 supported the concept of a specially prepared nurse clinician when it said:

'The baccalaureate programme should prepare the nurse for general professional nursing, the master's programme for specialization.'

Although the content of some of these early master's programmes was somewhat limited (nursing in particular was poorly defined and developed), the movement was towards a concept of clinical specialization.

Kohnke (1978), however, pointed out that 'the influence of medical specialization and the lack of clinical nursing supervision contributed to the development of the clinical specialist role'. She felt that in the early 1950s and before hospitals developed a more complicated bureaucratic system, the supervisor's roles were clinically oriented: 'their functions were those of master practitioner and, in hospitals containing schools of nursing, teacher'. As those supervisors and head nurses who were considered the nursing experts at that time became swamped with paper work and administrative duties, so they lost their clinical nursing skills. Added to this, as Kohnke (1978) pointed out, was the change in rewards for nursing from direct clinical involvement to managing the system. Whatever was the direct cause, greater specialization increased the administrative functions of supervisors and produced a change in the nursing care delivered (Christman, 1965).

Burd (1966), who traced the origin and development of the trend to specialization in American psychiatric nursing, saw it as a very old rather than new concept, and like De Witt (1900) she saw private duty nurses being identified as the early specialists who achieved their clinical abilities and reputation largely on their own, since there were then no formal courses for such work.

'When hospitals offered postgraduate courses the emphasis was on the work to be done rather than the study of an advanced level of practice.' (Burd, 1966)

Smoyak (1976) further supported Burd by stating:

'When the area is administration, teaching or supervision, the required courses are spelled out very clearly and given names and titles. But when nursing supposedly is the chief focus, the courses are simply listed as nursing (medical-surgical, psychiatric, and so on) or practicum or nursing major.'

Owing in part, therefore, to pressure from the national nursing associations to prepare clinical nurses as clinical nurse specialists, the universities developed courses at Master's degree level. The National League for Nursing (1952) reported 65 universities offering master's degree programmes in nursing, of which 90% offered some type of clinical specialist focus.

In the UK the development of degree programmes in nursing is a more recent event, and Manchester University was the first university where a clinical specialist option at master's degree level was available. Unfortunately only a very few nurses – fewer than five – took up this opportunity in the late 1970s and early 1980s. This was probably due to the low status of clinical nursing and the reluctance of managers to second clinical nurses to such courses.

'There has, in fact, been more debate about nurse education than any other subject over the years, and the thinking behind all the reports from Platt to Briggs to Project 2000, has been that the nurse must be free from at least part of her service commitment in order that she may learn more effectively.' (Whyte, 1977)

Briggs (DHSS, 1972) not only recognized the need for a new direction in nurse education but supported the development of clinical specialization:

'We consider, as we argued in Chapter VI, that clinical skills above the existing ward sister level should be recognized by enhanced status within the grade or by promotion to Nursing Officer within the same job as appropriate, by the creation of joint teaching, research and clinical posts and by the creation of special staff posts at various levels in, for instance, clinical research. This is a matter of the recognition of existing expertise and the development and recognition of new scope for expertise.'

The founding of the Joint Board of Clinical Nursing Studies in 1970 provided an increasing number of specialized advanced post-registration courses to meet the increasing demands and needs of nurse working with patients in specialized medical/surgical areas. According to Gardener (1976), 'Joint Board courses provide the opportunity to study a clinical specialty in depth'. It would appear from glancing over the considerable variety and number of them (37 in 1976), that they tended to follow medical specialities and in some instances emphasized the medical treatment, as shown in the comments made in a *Nursing Times* (1976) editorial referring to the renal course:

'Courses in renal nursing are approved only at centres where transplants are being done and this makes the course most interesting. In addition to working in the area where the dialysis is done you work in the wards associated with renal disease, as well as in the transplant wards.'

When introducing a new series on ten of the courses sponsored by the Joint Board of Clinical Nursing Studies, the *Nursing Mirror* (1976) editorial inferred that:

'with the emergence of the clinical nurse consultant and specialist, there is an added incentive to acquire specialist knowledge, for in addition to developing the basic skills, specialist training can now equip a nurse to develop her career at the bedside.'

Though Whyte (1977) described the founding of the Joint Board of Clinical Nursing Studies as 'a landmark in the history of nursing in this country', she made the point that:

'it is very important that these courses should be used properly, because the present link between the trained course member and her future patients is rather tenuous. At present those who do courses very often do not use the training, and those who do need training very often cannot be spared to take the course.'

However, for nurses who preferred to widen the scope of their work and make their careers in the clinical field, rather than move into administration or education, the need to develop specialist knowledge and skills, both in the community and hospital, was firmly supported by the Merrison Report (1979):

> 'Extended roles for nurses are developing as a result of specialization, for example, in renal dialysis, care of spinal injuries, and special care baby units. Advances in medical science often require parallel advances in nursing care, and nurses working closely with doctors are pioneering new roles. During our visit to North America we found a growing interest in the role of the clinical nurse specialist. The health departments told us of similar appointments in the UK, usually at nursing officer or ward sister level. Specialist nurses may also have an advisory or an executive function in a health district. The RCN submitted a list of posts showing the range of specialties which have developed. While we recognise the danger that specialization may lead to inflexibility, there is clearly a growing demand for specialist nursing skills in the care of certain groups of patients. We comment later on the need to reward special expertise, and on the preparation needed for advanced roles in nursing.'

National League for Nursing Education

In 1943 the National League for Nursing Education in North America appointed a committee on postgraduate clinical programmes to determine the basic principles for evaluation of clinical postgraduate courses, where students would study to become skilled bedside practitioners who would supervise clinical nursing services, teach in clinical nursing areas or serve as clinical nursing consultants (NLNE, 1943). Five clinical areas of concern were listed as being of major importance: psychiatric nursing, communicable disease nursing, tuberculosis nursing, obstetric nursing and paediatric nursing. The committee stressed that such courses would be university sponsored and situated in programmes in nursing education leading to a baccalaureate or higher degree (Brown, 1948).

With the beginning of their concern for the development of clinical specialization as a separate field, it noted that promotion in nursing careers almost invariably led away from patient care to teaching or administration. Also, training had not been sufficiently formalized so that any real distinction could be made between baccalaureate and master's degree course content in the newly developing master's level programmes.

Reports in the early 1950s spoke of the need for differentiating collegiate and more advanced nursing education, and for strengthening clinical graduate course content to emphasize nursing practice. For instance, Bridgman (1955), Dean of Skidmore College and advisor on nursing education to the Russell Sage Foundation, reported that:

> 'The few graduate courses exist to prepare clinical specialists and consultants in such areas as maternity and child care, care of the aged, medical-surgical nursing

and psychiatric nursing. Such courses should emphasize nursing in terms of the most comprehensive and skilled care of patients rather than nursing education or administration. They should include well planned, truly advanced clinical or field experience in the special type of nursing with accompanying instruction and guidance.'

Categorization of nursing specialties

Peplau (1965) identified ten possible categories (and sub-categories within them) for nursing specialization. This was a major step towards showing the fragmentation and diversity of opinion about such a development. The following is a breakdown of these ten specialty categories already in existence at that time:

(1) Organs and body systems, e.g. cardiac, renal, metabolic
(2) Age of the client, e.g. premature, juvenile, adolescent
(3) Degree of illness, e.g. acute, chronic, convalescent
(4) Length of illness, e.g. short term, intermediate, long term
(5) Nursing activities, e.g. medicine nurse, insulin nurse, blood nurse
(6) Fields of knowledge, e.g. nuclear nurse, autogenic, behaviourist nurse
(7) Sub-roles, e.g. mother surrogate, counsellor, health teacher
(8) Clinical services, e.g. obstetrics, paediatrics, surgery
(9) Professional goal, e.g. rehabilitation nurse, infection control nurse
(10) Area of practice, e.g. public health nurse, psychiatric, tuberculosis nurse

Rogers (1973), commenting on these categories and the possible increase in them, said:

'Nursing will become an expanding conglomeration of piecemeal specialties unless guidelines of some sort can be introduced for direction.'

Psychiatric nursing

When Peplau was developing the first master's programme to prepare clinical specialists in 1954, she found from her enquiries that people wanted both a traditional generalist and a super nurse to fix all psychiatry's ills. The National League for Nursing, commenting on the education of the clinical specialist in *Psychiatric Nursing* in 1958, said:

'The purpose of the clinical specialist in psychiatric nursing remains clear: to bring about advances in the art and science of psychiatric nursing and to promote the application of new knowledge and methods in the care of patients.'

It would seem that what nurses or psychiatric nurses do, or learn to do, in any given country has much to do with prevailing definitions of what is called 'mental illness', and of definitions of the nature of the corrective professional work that is needed to put patients in the direction of 'mental health'. As Peplau (1978) said:

> 'The dilemma of nurses and psychiatric nurses is clear. No basic or post-basic nursing programme can teach all possible theories used by psychiatrists in their work.'

If, therefore, there is not the time, or it is difficult to select which theoretical framework to teach in full, the content of the early education of the psychiatric nurse is in question. There is considerable difference in the type of tasks which nurses undertake in general hospitals as opposed to those in psychiatric settings: for example, in general hospitals nurses are bathing, feeding and toileting patients, whereas in psychiatric hospitals many patients carry out these activities for themselves. Peplau (1978) defined the work of nurses in psychiatric settings in two ways:

> '(a) as manager of the routines of life on a unit with kindness, but only a modicum of unselected theory; or
> (b) as a change agent who uses substantial theory to guide nurse interactions with patients with the aim of evoking substantial change in patient behaviour.'

As Clark (1967) stressed:

> 'The present structure of nursing in Britain demands that if a successful nurse wishes to advance beyond the grade of ward sister or charge nurse she must devote all her energies to either administration or teaching and forget about contributing directly to patient care, i.e. clinical work.'

Clark (1967) supported these comments and, following a visit sponsored by the Edwina Mountbatten Trust to a variety of psychiatric hospitals in the UK and elsewhere in Europe to see whether in fact there was discontent and a need to develop a clinical role for trained nurses, made several important observations. First, because nurses were inflexible in changing their functions and becoming independent practitioners in their own right, the 'vacuum' caused by this failure 'has been filled with people not specifically trained for a role of providing continuous care for psychiatric patients'. Secondly, large numbers of well educated and promising trained nurses had left because of:

> '(a) lack of fulfilment in the job itself;
> (b) lack of any readily discernible satisfying career opportunities; and
> (c) lack of any real nursing in those opportunities that were discernible.'

Perhaps a good example of this type of frustration and need for some sort of continued clinical contact was Cheadle's (1970) experiences as a community psychiatric nurse/social worker:

'The nurse has a role to play in the community; whether you call him a social worker or not is immaterial. I found the experience of seeing the patient's background at first hand immensely valuable in understanding him and what he requires both inside and outside hospital.'

Nurse-therapists

Psychiatric nurse-therapists have been seen as a great success in developing the clinical role of the nurse. Marks *et al.* (1977) described three years of operational research with clinical nurse specialists at the Bethlem Royal and Maudsley Hospitals from 1972 to 1975. There is no doubt that these nurse-therapists were successfully used in the treatment of such things as phobic and obsessive compulsive disorders, social anxieties and social skills deficits, and a variety of habit disorders. The three main advantages of using nurses as therapists rather than using psychiatrists or psychologists was put by Marks *et al.* (1976) as:

(1) The lower cost and shorter training of nurses compared to psychiatrists and psychologists.
(2) Less strain on teaching and administrative facilities. 'Psychiatric nursing could expand to meet the need for more therapists with less distortion of its present pattern of resources than could any other health care group.'
(3) A wider scope for recruitment in the general population. 'There are many more people with O levels than with A levels plus a university degree.'

It was also claimed by Marks and others that despite the monetary saving to the country, nurse-therapists fulfilled a new and valuable therapeutic function making important contributions to the teaching of their nursing colleagues and other professionals.

Wilson-Barnett (1976) and Duberley (1976) both criticized nurse-therapists as 'psychologists' assistants', and not clinical nurse specialists in their own right. Millar (1976), replying to this criticism, said:

'Nurse-therapists receive patient referrals from a wide variety of sources, not solely from psychiatrists, and they function independently of psychologists, so it would be grossly improper not to recognize them as nurse specialists with a specifically clinical role.'

The National Association for Mental Health (1977), reporting in the *Nursing Times*, urged more training for nurses in psychotherapy because it believed that 'psychotherapy has become a boom industry widely practised by quacks and charlatans, and that trained nurses in the community as well as in the hospital could help to protect the weak and vulnerable from exploitation.'

One advantage of having nurse-therapists in the community rather than in a hospital setting was put forward by Millar (1977). He suggested that they shortened the chain of referrals before treatment and limited excessive expenditure of money and time for the client.

Liaison nurse

In the USA the development of liaison nursing as a discipline which provides for a highly skilled level of co-ordination between the department of psychiatry and the general hospital is an interesting expansion in the role of the psychiatric nurse. Robinson (1974) felt that such a person brought their expertise into the general hospital 'to provide care for the mentally disturbed patient suffering from a physical illness and also to aid the patient who develops an iatrogenic illness brought on by the stress of disability and hospitalisation'.

It would seem that the title of 'liaison nurse' varied from institution to institution, but whatever they were called – clinical specialist, psychiatric nurse clinician or psychiatric nurse co-ordinator – this individual nurse played a significant role in assisting the patient suffering from some emotional problem. Robinson (1974), commenting on seven years' experience of this service, said that 'the liaison nurse has been accepted and has integrated her work into the hospital structure'. One liaison nurse would see an average of six patients each week, acting on the medical wards as a consultant in such specialties as intensive care and coronary care, and on the surgical wards in such specialties as paediatrics and neurology.

It was not until the late 1950s and early 1960s that liaison services began to appear. Some of the early and most effective efforts were conducted at the John Hopkins Hospital under Doctors Meyers and Mendelsoh. The introduction of the clinical nursing specialist into liaison psychiatry, however, was a gradual event and, as Robinson (1974) pointed out:

'Like most trends in nursing this one has developed in parallel fashion to the medical model, partially as a result of the consumer's need for expanded services and partially out of the nursing profession's desire to understand and utilise new technology.'

The work of the liaison nurse involves making an assessment of the patient and their environment, looking for stressors which may be causing the anxiety expressed through maladaptive behaviour. The main objective of the treatment or therapy is to either alter the nature of the stressor or to alter the means by which the patient deals with it. Liaison nursing appears highly specialized, drawing on knowledge from sociology, psychiatry, psychiatric nursing and a good understanding of the patient's physical disease.

Perhaps a similar innovation to liaison nursing was described by Biddulph (1976), where a psychiatric nurse in charge of a university department of psychiatry of 20 beds, with a day hospital attached, was given the opportunity of extending her role. This involved increasing the trained staff of her unit so that she could provide a consultancy service to nurses in the teaching hospital, a 700 bedded general hospital situated a quarter of a mile from the psychiatric unit. Unfortunately, in the absence of organized research there is no support or clarification of Biddulph's statement that 'initially, the requests were for assistance with disturbed and confused patients, but this has gradually changed to "teach me how to manage the patient".' Biddulph did go on to state, however, that:

'Our psychiatric nurse member saw her own role changing, her teaching function increasing, and her clinical skills used more in problem solving situations. The clinical content and pattern of care in the unit placed greater emphasis on community care and the identification of the patient's nursing, material and social needs.'

Mental handicap nursing

When discussing the therapeutic role of the nurse in caring for the mentally handicapped in hospital, Barker (1977) made a plea for the development of a specialized role:

'Nurses want to be recognized as specialists rather than patronized as "qualified custodians".'

Barker sees this specialist role 'based upon the practical and scientifically valid footing of behaviourism'.

Lee and Farrell (1975), commenting on the staff wastage and poor status attributed to the nursing of the mentally handicapped, would have liked to see the title 'nurse' changed to something like 'mental health practitioner' and the contents of the syllabus of training changed even further so that:

'The syllabus should be expanded to contain more of physical and mental development, psychology, psychiatry and aspects of sociology pertinent to the care of the mentally handicapped, as well as a grounding in physical care.'

Psychogeriatric nursing care

If it seems that the field of mental handicap nursing was finding it difficult to develop its own specialist role, there was an interesting development in psychogeriatric care, considered another low status area in
nursing in the UK. Leopold *et al.* (1975) discussed a 12 month progress
report on the work of a clinical nursing officer appointed to the community psychiatric nursing service in the Isis Group of Hospitals. In broad
terms, the clinical nursing officer 'was to link more closely together the
psychiatric hospital and community services for the elderly and become
a working member of both'. There was no rigid job description and the
nurse was given the flexibility to work from a broad framework of
'assessment, domiciliary nursing care, multi-disciplinary team work,
nurse consultancy service, and training and education rather than the
customary enumerated detailed work directives'. The result of this project appears to have been very successful with the nursing officer's role
developing into one of a liaison officer.

Peplau (1978) felt that the future of psychiatric nurses depended on:

'(1) The competence brought to the work as a consequence of basic or post-basic
    nursing education.
 (2) The definition of mental illness and, therefore, of the work of "mentally ill"
    patients, that prevails in a given setting.
 (3) The extent of consensus around the question of whether each profession
    should or should not have only discrete, unique, circumscribed roles or
    whether there can be overlap (as, for example, in talking with patients,
    which all professions do), and if so, to what extent (i.e. only counselling,
    counselling and the various psychotherapies).
 (4) The cost of certain kinds of care (e.g. psychotherapy), the difference in
    status and salary levels (e.g. physicians, nurses, etc.), and the numbers of
    persons needed and available to provide certain kinds of care may also be
    countervailing or influential factors.'

Medical involvement and specialization in nursing

Between 1974 and 1977 the *British Medical Journal* organized three interesting discussions on:

(1) New alternatives in the National Health Service (BMJ, 1974)
(2) Medical manpower (BMJ, 1976)
(3) Clinical responsibility (BMJ, 1977)

With regard to the first of these, the topics included: conditions which
general practitioners could treat at home, how the community could cope

with discharged patients, and whether nurses would take more clinical responsibility if given it.

Flindall (1974) pointed out in her contribution to the conference that 'nurses have proved willing and able to take clinical responsibility, yet even where this occurs it is not openly acknowledged but hidden under the doctor's responsibility'. In the discussion which followed it was suggested that if more nurses were trained to the level of the midwife, who already made a clinical diagnosis, or the intensive care sister who accepted 'tremendous clinical responsibility', then it might result in the need for 'fewer doctors' and a 'rationalization' of health care delivery.

In the second discussion session, in 1976 on 'medical manpower and how much can ancillaries take over', the development in psychiatry of nurse-therapists was highlighted. Bhate (1976) suggested that 'instead of importing immigrant doctors, why not spend some money training carefully chosen nurses as therapists'. It was further pointed out that perhaps the most important factor in determining the extent to which nurses can do tasks traditionally performed by doctors was the individual nurse's attitudes and personality.

The third discussion session, in 1977 with regard to 'clinical responsibility', led Winder (1977) to state that:

'Doctors became bored with routine, uneventful dialysis, and wanted to have more time for the other clinical aspects of nephrology, as well as research. This change led to nurses becoming highly specialized in the skills of dialysis treatment and for technicians trained in the management of the machinery to play a larger part.'

Winder went on to point out that although the specialist nurse in dialysis work was an expert in a small field, it was the physician who was able to offer a far greater range of knowledge and understanding with regard to a patient's treatment. In the discussion which followed, stress was placed on the importance of treating nurses as 'separate but equal to doctors', and that doctors should be pleased to see the 'growing professionalism' of the people who worked with them, because it gave doctors more 'opportunity to move on and do other things'.

Specialization in medicine and the delegation of medical tasks

At a joint symposium in 1974 between the five Royal Colleges of Nursing, Midwives, Surgeons, Physicians and Obstetricians and Gynaecologists, to discuss current problems, the most striking factor to emerge from the discussions was the need for a better career structure for the clinical nurse,

and the resentment by doctors at the nurses' breakaway from their traditional role as handmaidens to the medical profession. In an article in *The
Times*, Gillie (1975a), commenting on the Merrison Report (1975), stated that:

> 'We will never be able to train sufficient doctors to supply demand unless we
> rethink what jobs doctors should be doing. Doctors could be used much more
> efficiently if the nurses were allowed to do more, and were paid to do more.'

In 1975, the British Medical Association predicted that there would be a
critical shortage of doctors within two or three years. They saw as contributory factors at that time the failure of many foreign doctors to pass
new language and competence tests and the expected emigration of British
doctors to better paid jobs in Europe when the Common Market restrictions
were lifted. It is perhaps interesting to note that the shortage of doctors,
especially junior doctors and general practitioners, has been a worrying
trend in the UK in the 1990s.

In an article in *The Sunday Times*, however, Gillie (1975b) pointed out that
a new type of nurse – a 'nurse consultant' – could fill this gap and that such
a person, among other responsibilities, could teach medical students and
make medical rounds. He indicated that there had been interesting
examples where nurses had taken on specialized roles, for example in
family planning and psychiatry, where it would appear that according to
medical opinion alone such innovations have been very successful.

Miller and Backett (1980) found that over two thirds of a random sample
of 690 general practitioners in the UK were in favour of the extended role
and were prepared to delegate clinical tasks to a nurse. Bowling (1980)
researched the attitudes of nurses in general practice towards taking over
such medical tasks from the doctors and found a wide range of contradictory views reflecting continuing uncertainty about the nurse's role.

The British Medical Journal (BMJ, 1978) summed up the situation in an
editorial:

> 'How far the clinical nurse will help in primary care in Britain in the next decade
> is a matter for doctors, nurses and patients to judge ... It is not simply a matter of
> diagnostic tests, operating theatres, or laboratories. Techniques have their place
> in medicine, but the essential feature of medical practice is that someone who is
> ill, or thinks he is ill, seeks the advice of a doctor whom he trusts. All else in the
> practice of medicine derives from this consultation, and any discussion about
> extending the role of the clinical nurse must recognize this central fact.'

Unfortunately, many nurses have traditionally seen themselves as extensions of the doctor's therapeutic functions and the unique role of the nurse
has been lost sight of. It would seem, therefore, that in certain situations
doctors are handing over tasks to nurses and technicians. The reasons for
this development could be the result of increasing specialization and

advancement in medical science or the shortages of medical manpower due to financial constraints.

Early definitions of the clinical nurse specialist

In order to establish a definition of the clinical nurse specialist Baker and Kramer (1970) set up an interview survey of the directors of nursing in 37 medical centres in the USA, plus six nurse graduates in each centre. For the purposes of their study, they defined a clinical nurse specialist as 'an individual prepared in nursing at the master's level and not assigned to a specific patient unit, i.e. not listed on the ward time roster, but responsible for and actively engaged in planning and giving care'.

Any nurse who fitted this definition was considered to be a clinical nurse specialist, even if her job included additional duties such as overall administrative responsibility. From the preliminary interviews, three main areas emerged that seemed suitable for further investigation by Baker and Kramer. They were:

'(1) The appropriateness and meaningfulness of the title for the nurse in this role
(2) The role functions of the clinical nurse specialist
(3) The source and scope of authority within the organization for nurses in this position.'

Interestingly, those directors of nursing who expressed difficulties in placing this job title within their existing organized structure, either created new positions or employed the clinical nurse specialist in an available position, usually at the supervisory level, while expecting and instructing him/her to evolve activities consistent with the clinical nurse specialist's role. Confusion over the title was evident in those organizations in which both academically prepared nurses and experienced nurses without advanced education were employed in the clinical nurse specialist role. Much of the literature supported Baker and Kramer's findings on the variety of role functions which were given to clinical nurse specialists. The strongest theme, supported by Simms (1966) and Reiter (1966), was that the clinical nurse specialist should function as an expert practitioner and role model. Pohl (1965) and Harrington and Theis (1968) supported the teaching, change-agent, and co-ordinating function of the specialist, and to a lesser extent Yokes (1966), Wald and Leonard (1964) and Peplau (1965) saw research and the counsellor roles as important.

Baker and Kramer (1970) found that all the directors of nursing expressed some concern with regard to the clinical nurse specialist's position in the organizational structure: 'Line placement has the advantage of a circumscribed area of control and a positional source of authority', whereas 'staff placement has the advantage of greater mobility and self-selection of patients for care'. From Baker and Kramer's research into a satisfying definition for the clinical nurse specialist and the way to ensure positive results from employing such an individual, three recommendations were made:

'(1)   Clearly defined job activities known and understood by herself and others
(2)   A title consonant with her functions
(3)   Knowledge that she has the authority to take action that will lead to changes.'

Hellman (1974), in giving her definition of a clinical nurse specialist, believed that such a person should be prepared at the master's degree level, and that 'quality of health care' was of utmost importance. She gave a list of functions of the specialist which included: expert practitioner, role model, change agent, teacher, researcher and consultant. In concluding, Hellman (1974) said:

'The role of the clinical nurse specialist is a flexible one, and must have a flexible definition. The generalities of the role can be defined and communicated, and they express the commonalities among all such practitioners, regardless of specialty. But the specifics of the role can only be defined in the context of the individual practitioner in her particular setting and in her time.'

The American Nurses' Association (ANA, 1976) issued an operational definition of the clinical nurse specialist:

'A practitioner holding a master's degree with a concentration in specific areas of clinical practice. The role of the clinical nurse specialist is defined by the needs of a select client (patient, family and/or community) population, the expectations of the larger society, and the clinical expertise of the nurse. By exercising judgement and demonstrating leadership ability the clinical nurse specialist functions within a field of practice that focuses on the needs of the client system and encompasses interaction with others in the nursing and health care systems serving the client. The clinical nurse specialist role includes participation in activities designed to continue self-development, advance the goals of the nursing profession, and promote effective collaborative relationships with members of other health care disciplines.'

From this definition three major requirements appear to be significant in defining the clinical nurse specialist's role:

(1)   A registered nurse holding a master's degree in nursing with an emphasis on clinical nursing
(2)   One who demonstrates a high degree of competence

(3)   One who works closely in a collegial and collaborative way with other health care team members.

The Registered Nurses' Association of Ontario, in a statement in 1976, defined the role of the clinical nurse specialist in a similar manner:

'A registered nurse with a master's degree in a clinical nursing specialty who is accountable for providing a high quality of nursing care and for improving standards of health care. The primary functions of the clinical nurse specialist are to give direct nursing care to patients and families when specialized expertise is required, and to influence others to improve nursing care. The role of the clinical nurse specialist includes the functions of practitioner, consultant, educator, change agent and researcher.'

Royal College of Nursing of the United Kingdom

The commitment by the Royal College of Nursing (RCN) to the development of a clinical career structure for nurses and the concept of the clinical nurse specialist goes back to 1970 when Richard Crossman, the then Secretary of State for Social Services, appointed a Committee on Nursing (Briggs) to review the role of the nurse and midwife in the hospital and the community, and the education and training required. The recommendations by the RCN working party to the Briggs Committee were supported. For example, in 1971 a motion was put forward:

'That this meeting of the RCN Representative Body strongly supports the recommendations in the RCN evidence to the Committee on Nursing that an advanced clinical role for the nurse/midwife be identified by the creation of posts of nurse/midwife consultant.'

Although the Committee on Nursing made no specific recommendations in respect of the establishment of a clinical specialist grade, it did recognize the level of clinical ability and responsibility of some ward sisters:

'Ward sisters of higher clinical skills, often in specialized fields, may already exercise advisory functions to other nurses and members of other professions, and this kind of development should be encouraged.' (para. 541)

The need for research into the role of clinical nurse specialists was supported by the Briggs Report (DHSS, 1972) when it said: 'This is a matter of the recognition of existing expertise and the development and recognition of new scope for expertise.' (para. 684) Lack of this necessary research data may account for the continuing appearance of resolutions at the RCN Representative Body meetings. In 1977 two motions were carried:

(1) 'To request the DHSS immediately to undertake a study of the role and career structure of the clinical nurse.'
(2) 'To formulate and negotiate a salary and career structure for those engaged in clinical nursing complementary to that which exists for nurse managers and nurse educators.'

In October 1975 the RCN held a seminar at Leeds Castle in Kent to study the subject of the clinical nurse specialist (RCN, 1975). Kerrane (1975), reporting on the proceedings for the *Nursing Mirror*, made the following points:

'The average ward sister is unable to fill the expectations of the role (of clinical specialist) because of increasing pressures and her responsibility for areas other than direct patient care. The nursing officer and clinical teacher grades might conceivably be developed into specialist roles, but a total restructuring of their responsibilities would be needed.'

Duberley (1976), however, disagreed with this assumption and put forward a case for the ward sister acting as the clinical nurse specialist. Referring to Georgopoulos and Christman's (1970) study where three clinical nurse specialists functioned as ward sisters, improving direct patient care, Duberley said:

'Direction and supervision of patient care is perhaps more acceptable from the clinical nurse specialist functioning in the capacity of ward sister than as a staff consultant.'

Ashworth (1975), however, believed that to achieve continuity and completeness of care there must be nurses who were not confined to one ward or department, but who were free to follow (or precede) patients where necessary from home to hospital and vice versa, who could be consulted by nurses anywhere who felt that they could help to solve patient care problems, and who could provide knowledgeable advice to nursing management or other bodies. Supporting the need for another kind of nurse with greater depth and breadth of educational preparation and scope, Ashworth agreed with the other participants of the Leeds Castle seminar group when she said that 'ultimately a university education such as the MSc (nursing option) course offered at Manchester University would be the appropriate preparation'. The financial and educational implications of all ward sisters achieving an MSc degree in nursing was seen as unrealistic at that time but there was strong support for Ashworth's views.

Castledine (1977) argued, however, that because of the excessive demands made on the ward sisters by such things as growth of knowledge, extended role functions of the trained nurse, teaching commitments and increase in managerial responsibilities, perhaps the ward sister should be replaced by someone else (a clinical consultant) who would have direct responsibility for leading and carrying out patient care with a team which is not necessarily ward or departmentally based. This would leave the co-ordinating functions and administrative responsibilities of patient and ward care in the hands of someone else; for example, the nurse manager or 'patient care co-ordinator' envisaged and tried out by the McMaster University Medical Center. McPhail (1978), in describing the role of these patient care co-ordinators, showed how nursing authority had lost its hierarchical nature and become decentralized with direct power and responsibility for problems being in the hands of the people on the unit or ward. The patient care co-ordinator had a multitude of responsibilities, one of which was to call in the clinical specialist when necessary for patient care and staff development.

The report of the first RCN working party on the need for advanced clinical posts appeared to have some problems in separating clinical nurse specialist from clinical nurse consultant:

'The title of clinical nurse specialist (or consultant) is not important provided that it is descriptive of a function and identifies the nurse holding a post as a clinical expert.'

It is difficult to determine at what point a clinical nurse specialist would become a clinical nurse consultant, because this would probably depend on his/her knowledge, experience and amount of consultation with other health workers including doctors. The Leeds Castle seminar report (RCN, 1975) did not help much in clarifying the position: 'The development of a clinical nurse specialist/consultant involved identifying not one role but certainly two, and perhaps more.' Nor did it give much idea of who these specialist nurses were, or what type of nursing decisions they were making.

Ashworth (1975) did, however, follow the American patterns and pointed to the following as the main elements of the role of the clinical nurse specialist:

'(1) Director of care
(2) Co-ordinator
(3) Change agent
(4) Teacher
(5) Consultant to colleagues
(6) Researcher to colleagues.'

In its evidence to the Royal Commission on the National Health Service the RCN (1977) pointed out:

'There is a need to identify new roles for nurses as specialists and consultants, in different spheres of practice ... nurses aspiring to fill these new roles would need to have studied to increase their knowledge and to have had considerable experience in the particular specialty. Special courses of preparation would be necessary; the nurse consultant would require preparation in greater depth than the nurse specialist.'

Early clinical nurse specialists in the UK

Apart from the nurse-therapists and other developments in psychiatric nursing described earlier, there are several accounts and references to so-called clinical nurse specialists in the UK.

The first appointment of an infection control sister was made at the Torbay Hospital and described by Gardener and others in the *Lancet* (1974). Three key elements emerged as significant in this development:

'(1)   The collection and recording of information relevant to infection control
(2)   Extensive liaison with professional groups in hospital, and
(3)   The organising and carrying out of bacteriological surveys under the direction of the control of infection officer and consultant bacteriologist.'
(Grant, 1970)

O'Connor (1971), describing the work of Ruth Seddon, a nursing officer at Dudley Road Hospital, Birmingham, referred to 'a new breed of nurses specializing in the field of infection control'. Seddon, talking about this development, said that 'there are no fancy reasons for my interest in infection control, it has to do with patient care'. She further pointed out that her work involved keeping records, making ward surveys, teaching, research, and working closely with other health workers. With regard to why such a post should be occupied by a nurse, Seddon stated, 'I think it is true that you have to be a nurse for nurses to accept you and you have to be a sister for consultants to talk to you'. Parker (1976), referring to a clinical nurse consultant in infection control, felt that 'the special contribution of the nurse is her experience in all aspects of patient care. It is nurses who carry out, or prepare for, most of the procedures to which patients are subjected'. Parker showed that knowledge of the specialized field, careful monitoring, patient involvement, co-ordination or nursing control measures, research, teaching, advanced training and education were essential aspects of the clinical nurse consultant in infection control. She pointed out, however, that not all nurses working in this field fulfilled the role of clinical nurse consultant.

Developments in surgery, leaving patients with a colostomy, ileostomy or a urinary diversion, led to a gradual appearance of nurses as specialists in stoma care. Saunders was the leader in this field of care at St Bartholomew's Hospital in the early 1970s. At a stoma care symposium, Morgans (1975) argued the case for a nurse to be involved with such work:

'This working party looked at other possibilities within the community and at other people we could involve, but we could find no one with all the expertise that we have and can give our patients.'

Saunders (1976), commenting on her role, felt that future stoma nurses should have some form of preparation as the role involves liaison with nursing, medical and associated staff involved with the patient, giving direct psychological and physical support to the patient, teaching, keeping statistics, and keeping up to date with new developments in stoma care. The *Lancet* (1974), commenting on the approval of two Joint Board courses for nurses to become stoma therapists, supported the enterprise and looked forward to 'others forms of nurse expert' developing.

Perhaps the development of a clinical nurse specialist in anaesthetics was the answer to the growing concern expressed by many about the future of the nurse in the operating theatre. Millington (1976) believed that 'wherever a patient is receiving medical care, so must there be a nurse. Whether that patient is conscious or unconscious, he still needs nursing care.' A small scale study carried out by Heggarty and Kirchner (1977) involved a questionnaire and interview with anaesthetists and anaesthetic nurses of different grades. The majority supported the role of a specialized nurse in the anaesthetic area. One significant finding also was that:

'Although reassurance, rapport and nursing care were rated joint first in order of priority of anaesthetic nurses' functions by anaesthetists, all anaesthetic nurses stated that these tasks took up least time during their work.'

Finally, it was felt that if anaesthetic nurses had 'a year's post-registration course and then made pre-operative visits, ran minor surgical lists (having been strictly assessed first), performed epidural "top-ups" and put intravenous infusions up in the wards, taught student nurses, etc.,' they would gain much more job satisfaction and feel more useful in their role.

This conclusion not only had implications for the future of anaesthetic nurses but for the future of the nurse's role in general. Stephens and Boaler (1977) conducted a questionnaire into the knowledge and attitudes of nurses caring for patients immediately after operation. They found that while this was a nursing responsibility, nurses were not adequately trained in the required techniques. The *Nursing Mirror* (1977) felt that the clinical nurse consultant, as put forward by Millington (1976), 'has an important role as a clinical teacher, particularly in this vulnerable area of post-operative management'. Millington (1976) found that a major part of her role involved pre- and post-operative patient counselling, and dealing with problems regarding equipment and techniques. Added to this, however, she felt that the role of clinical nurse consultant should be a 'staff' post, working in consultation with others and having a research and teaching function.

The role of a nurse consultant in child health was discussed by Cowper-Smith (1977). She pointed out the flexibility of such a post, 'moving around wards, corridors and departments, as well as going into the community'. Working from a newly created health education unit, this specially prepared nurse gave counselling and advice, contributed to clinical research, and worked in close consultation with other health workers.

Parkinson (1977) pointed out that the role of area nurse, child health, was:

'the first time that a nurse consultant had been appointed at a senior level whose clear responsibilities were those of an expert professional advisor. The role involves giving continuity to the school health services, participating and carrying out policies on screening, assessment and prophylactic measures and among those functions already stated providing an advisory role on child health to the area health authority.'

If the role of nurse specialist/consultant was well established in child health, Freeman (1975) made a case for nurse specialists in obstetric practice in the community. She said, '[if] continuity of care is lacking, that change is needed and desired. My suggestion is that a new specialist nursing role be created to take charge of ante- and postnatal care'. In support, Freeman held that communication between hospital and community frequently broke down, resulting in mothers not seeing the domiciliary midwife as soon as they should. Also that the rise in mother support groups showed that 'we are failing to provide a satisfactory obstetric service ... Postnatal depression and the increasing number of non-accidental injuries to babies and young children ... leaving mothers in need of support', were all contributory factors to the demand for better care.

The changing role of nurses in the management of diabetes led to the development of specialist nurses at St Thomas's Hospital in London. Judd *et al.* (1976) found that specialist nurses often gained the 'close confidence of many patients who may be unable to relax with a busy doctor'. It was also found that these nurses played a significant role in the education of the patient and of community nursing staff, thus providing a co-ordinator role in the care of the diabetic.

Just as nurses have developed their role in the management of diabetes, so they have extended their role in family planning. In 1974 a pilot study was carried out at King's College Hospital, London, with the help of an American nurse practitioner. Following a special training course, nine nurse specialists took over the management of a special experimental clinic. Their work involved making a medical examination, taking a history and discussing the choice of contraception, and according to Newton *et al.* (1977) 'this pilot experiment of nurse specialist work in family planning indicates that a logical extension of the nurse and midwife's role in family planning is possible'. Medical support for this development appeared in the *British Medical Journal* (Newton *et al.*, 1976).

Occupational health nurses have been very concerned with issues related to their scope of practice; for example, Jarman (1978) examined the extended role of her work and asked 'am I a doctor?' She referred to the health assessments, counselling and emergencies she dealt with in the scope of her practice. Added to this, she had to work alone without other professional support. It would seem from what Jarman said that there was a need for a study of the role of the occupational health nurse:

'There are no national guidelines or standards on what is good occupational health nursing practice, and although this allows for initiative, it also allows for much bad practice and waste of nursing skills.'

Although this may be looked on as a special case, other areas of clinical specialization should be examined to see if any of Jarman's comments apply.

There have been several attempts at implementing the role of a clinical nurse specialist. Biddulph (1976) referred, in an unpublished report, to the work of a senior ward sister with 20 years' experience in neurosurgical nursing. She was allowed to explore a role specializing in the care of patients with neurosurgical conditions and patients admitted to the hospital with head injuries. Martin (1975) talked about how she went to other wards in the hospital, visited other hospitals, and went to patients' homes when 'specialist advice and nursing care was needed'. It would seem that Martin provided expert care and advice not only to the patient but to those who were involved in the care; lack of research data, however, failed to confirm this.

In his annual report, Tiffany (1976), Director of Nursing at the Royal Marsden Hospital, referred to the development of clinical nurse specialists at the hospital. He said that 'the need for such a nurse arose out of the demand from experienced nurses who wanted to develop their clinical skills and continue to give direct patient care'.

Clinical specialists working at the Royal Marsden cover stoma care, infection control, nutrition, community liaison, the staging unit, mastectomy, and metabolic and intravenous therapy. More than any other innovation at the Royal Marsden, the establishment of an intravenous therapy team raised the most questions, for it meant nurses were now performing a procedure which had previously been the prerogative of the medical staff. Tiffany argued that what was a medical function one day – such as taking blood pressure – could be viewed as a skill basic to certain kinds of nursing care the next day. Also, he felt that 'contrary to popular belief the definition of what is a medical function and what is a nursing function is not a matter of law; where the law becomes involves at all it follows and legitimizes agreed practice'. How these clinical nurse specialists were accepted by ward sisters at the Royal Marsden was high-lighted by Cowper-Smith (1977), when she attended and reported on a special study at the hospital to discuss the problems. It would seem that some sisters viewed the specialist as having higher status, greater flexibility and prestige. With these developments at the Royal Marsden and else-where, it could be said that the role of the clinical nurse specialist was slowly growing out of existing structures because of recognized patient needs for more expert and specialized care, and by experienced nurses who wanted to stay in a direct relationship with patients.

Grabow (1978), Osborne (1978) and Rigby (1978) are three nurses who reported the nature of their work as a clinical nurse specialist at the Royal Marsden Hospital. All three worked in medically dominated specialties. Burdge (1978), however, had developed a clinical nursing officer role at the Royal Marsden which attempted to develop the suggestion put forward in the Salmon Report (MoH, 1966).

There are opportunities for nurses to concentrate on a particular clinical specialist field. Staying in these specialized areas does not necessarily involve becoming a clinical nurse specialist. Kratz (1976) said that there were 'specialists and specialists'. She argued that 'in order to qualify as a clinical nurse specialist it is of course necessary that the specialist should demonstrate not only that she acts recognisably as a nurse, but that she has specialist nursing knowledge.'

The Canadian experience

In October 1971, the Canadian Nurses' Association directors set up a three member task force to prepare a working paper on specialization in nursing (Canadian Nurses' Association, 1973), and they asked for comments. It was felt by the Association that clinical nursing specialization would be increasing over the next few years without adequate planning. Some of the questions agreed in the paper were:

'(1) What specialty fields should take priority in development?
(2) When is care by a specialist in the best interest of the patient and also an economically sound proposition?
(3) What training specifications should be set up for various kinds of specialties?
(4) Who will organize and provide this training?
(5) How will specialists be identified and recognized?'

With regard to the expanding role of the nurse, Anderson *et al.* (1975) said that 'nursing content should be at the core of education for nursing prac-titioners', and if this nursing framework was not developed, nurses working in specialized fields would be viewed as physicians' assistants.

Shortages of medical personnel in Canada resulted in growing demands on the health care system and similar approaches to those in America were made by Canadian physicians. As Hurd (1972) pointed out, however, this development met with resistance, particularly as some nurses felt that this would be going back to control of nurses by doctors. In 1973, the Canadian Nurses' Association issued the following statement on specialization in nursing:

'*Position*
In keeping with its goal of promoting the highest possible standards of nursing care, the Association recommends recognition of degrees or levels of speciali-zation within the profession.

Levels of Specialization
Two types of programme should be offered: post-diploma or post-basic and master's degree level.

Areas of Specialization
In the area of specialized care and services, priorities can only be established after identifying current nursing activities, reviewing health problems in Canada and assessing clients' needs.'

The first Canadian nurses to become clinical nurse specialists had American role models and American education, therefore it could be said that they followed the American model very closely. In doing this, however, the introduction of Canadian clinical nurse specialists was kept deliberately at a low key, according to Cahoon (1975). This was to avoid exaggerated expectations and to allow slow implementation. Darcovich (1973) appeared to support these comments when she said, 'There is no one, clearly defined role for the clinical nurse specialist'. She went on to point out, however, that there were two streams of development, 'one primarily involving direct patient care, and the other primarily involving staff education'. However, the Registered Nurses' Association of Ontario, in a statement in 1976, felt that the role of the clinical nurse specialist included the functions of practitioner, consultant, educator, change agent and researcher.

Developments in other countries

In many other countries besides the USA and Canada, an advanced clinical role for nurses developed because of shortages of medical manpower. For example, in Zimbabwe, Fraser Ross (1975) described how advanced clinical nurses were used successfully in two ways: first, by 'assisting a medical practitioner in the work of running his hospital and so releasing him for those duties for which he is more highly trained'; secondly, by 'staffing rural hospitals and district hospitals were medical practitioners visit on a regular basis'. By taking on these two functions it appeared that the nurses were performing functions normally undertaken by doctors and making medical decisions when they were placed in isolated rural situations.

Katz *et al.* (1976) described a two year study carried out in Australia, the purpose of which was to discover the opinions of nurses, doctors and patients regarding the roles, tasks, functions and skills that nurses were performing and would perform in the future. The results of this study indicated that a strong case existed for more responsibility to be given to nurses with regard to health care. It was found, for instance, that nurses could perform certain medical tasks as well as doctors and that patients accepted nurses functioning in this way. Katz argued that, 'by fusing nursing skills with newly acquired medical tasks, patients will receive a type of care best described as an intermingling of the cure and care components'.

Of course, the question is should nurses be the physician's assistant, moving into those areas which the medical profession is too easily willing to give up? Katz believed that nursing would be 'widened, enriched and enhanced' if it developed in this way. However, it is debatable whether such extensions are desirable and whether they help to clarify the purpose and definition of what constitutes nursing care.

References

Abel-Smith, B. (1960) *A History of the Nursing Profession.* Heinemann, London.

ANA (1976) *The Scope of Nursing Practice.* Document May 1976, chaired by I.G. Mauksch. American Nurses' Association.

Anderson, J., Marcus, A.M., Gemeroy, H., Perry, F. & Campperman (1975) *The Canadian Nurse*, **71** (9), 34-5.

Ashworth, P.A. (1975) The clinical nurse consultant. *Nursing Times*, **71** (15), 574-7.

Austin, R. (1977) Sex and gender in the future of nursing I and II. *Nursing Times Occasional Papers*, **73** (34), 113-16 and **73** (35), 117-20.

Baker, C. & Kramer, M. (1970) To define or not to define: the role of the clinical specialist. *Nursing Forum*, **4** (1), 45-55.

Barker, P. (1977) Jack-of-all-trades nurse with a specialty in custodial care. *Health and Social Service Journal*, **87** (4536), 666-7.

Bendall, E. (1976) Learning for reality. *Journal of Advanced Nursing*, **1** (1), 309.

Bendall, E. (1977) The future of British nurse education. *Journal of Advanced Nursing*, **2** (2), 171-81.

Bhate, S. (1976) Two streams of nurses – discussion. *British Medical Journal*, No. 6000, Vol. 1, 3 January, p. 28.

Biddulph, C. (1976) The clinical specialist. *Nurses and Health Care*, pp. 43-5. King Edward's Hospital Fund for London.

Bowling, P.A. (1980) To do or not to do? *Nursing Mirror*, **151** (3), 30-32.

Bridgman, G. (1955) In *New Directions in Patient Centred Nursing* (ed. Abdellah *et al.*) (1973). Macmillan, New York.

BMJ (1974) New alternatives in the NHS. How many doctors do we need? *British Medical Journal* No. 5941, Vol. **4**, 16 November, 389–93.

BMJ (1976) Medical manpower: I. How much can ancillaries take over? *British Medical Journal* No. 6000, Vol. **1**, 3 January, 25–30.

BMJ (1977) Clinical responsibility. *British Medical Journal* No. 6102, Vol. **2**, 17 December, 1584–9.

BMJ (1978) Extending the role of the clinical nurse. *British Medical Journal*, No. 6148, Vol. **2**, 11 November, 1320.

Brown, E.L. (1948) *Nursing for the Future.* Russell Sage Foundation, New York.

Burd, S. (1966) *The Clinical Specialisation Trend in Psychiatric Nursing.* Rutgers State University Graduate School of Education, unpublished doctoral dissertation, New Brunswick.

Burdge, L. (1978) The role of the clinical nursing officer. *Nursing Times,* **74** (31), 1299–1300.

Cahoon, M. (1975) The Canadian experience. In: *New Horizons in Clinical Nursing.* Royal College of Nursing, London.

Canadian Nurses' Association (1973) *Discussion paper on Specialisation in Nursing.* Prepared for the Canadian Nurses' Association by Alice J. Baumgart. Canadian Nurses' Association, Ontario.

Castledine, G. (1977) Report of the RCN Association of Nursing Practice Annual Conference – Charge Nurse Drops Bombshell over the Future of Ward Sisters. *Nursing Mirror,* **144**, 29 September, 3.

Cheadle, J. (1970) The psychiatric nurse as a social workers. *Nursing Times,* **66**, 26 November, 1520–2.

Christman, L. (1965) The influence of specialisation on the nursing profession. *Nursing Science,* **3** (6), 446–53.

Clark, M.A. (1967) A clinical role for senior nurses in social psychiatry. *International Journal of Nursing Studies,* **4**, 331–40.

Cowper-Smith, F. (1977) Why does the nurse specialist threaten sister? *Nursing Times,* **73** (50), 1942–3.

Darcovich, O. (1973) Spotlight on the clinical nurse specialist. *The Canadian Nurse,* **69** (9), 42.

De Witt, K. (1900) Specialist in nursing. *American Journal of Nursing (Practical Points on Private Nursing Department),* **1** (14), 17.

DHSS (1972) *Report of the Committee on Nursing.* Chairman, Professor Asa Briggs. CMNB 5115. HMSO, London.

Duberley, J. (1976) The clinical nurse specialist. *Nursing Times,* **72** (46), 1794–5.

Flindall, J. (1974) Would nurses take clinical responsibility if given it? *British Medical Journal,* **4**, 16 November, 392–3.

Fraser Ross, W. (1975) The advanced clinical nurse (ACN) and the health team. *Central African Journal of Medicine,* **21** (11), 243–5.

Freeman, M. (1975) Maternity nurse practitioner. *Nursing Times,* **71** (47), 1853–7.

Gardener, M.G. (1976) Courses in clinical nursing. *Nursing Mirror,* **143** (5), 45–7.

Georgopoulos, B.G. & Christman, L. (1970) The clinical nurse specialist: a role model. In: *The Clinical Nurse Specialist.* American Journal of Nursing Company, New York.

Gillie, O. (1975a) Where nurses can be doctors. *The Times,* 20 April.

Gillie, O. (1975b) Plan for nurse consultants to fill doctor gap. *Sunday Times,* 14 September.

Grabow, R. (1978) The staging unit. *Nursing Times,* **74** (28), 1168–9.

Grant, M.L. (1970) Infection control sister. *Nursing Times,* **66** (21), 659–60.

Harrington, H. & Theis, C. (1968) Institutional factors perceived by baccalaureate graduates as influencing their performances. *Nursing Research,* **17**, 338.

Heggarty, J.M. & Kirchner, G.B. (1977) The British anaesthetic nurse – her role and future. *Nursing Mirror,* **145** (14), 25–7.

Hellman, C. (1974) The making of a clinical specialist. *Nursing Outlook,* **22**, March, 165–7.

Hurd, J.L. (1972) Directional signals for nursing's expanding role. *The Canadian Nurse,* **68** (1), 21–35.

Jarman, B.M. (1978) The extending role of the British occupational health nurse. Doctor? Safety worker? Nurse? *Journal of Advanced Nursing,* **3** (2), 189–98.

Judd, S.A., O'Leary, E., Read, P. & Fox, C. (1976) The changing role of nurses in the management of diabetes. *British Journal of Hospital Medicine,* **16** (3), 251–5.

Katz, F.M., Mathews, K., Pepe, T. & White, R.H. (1976) *Stepping Out.* University Press Ltd, New South Wales.

Kerrane, T.A. (1975) The clinical nurse specialist. *Nursing Mirror,* **140**, 30 January, 63–5.

Kohnke, M. (1978) *The Case for Consultation in Nursing Designs for Professional Practice.* J. Wiley & Sons, New York.

Kratz, C. (1976) The clinical nurse consultant. *Nursing Times,* **72** (46), 1792–3. First printed in the *Queen's Nursing Journal,* October 1976, **19** (7).

Lancet (1974) Stoma-therapy specialists (editorial). *Lancet,* **1**, 9 February, 204.

Lee, H. & Farrell, P. (1975) Mental health practitioner? *Nursing Times,* **71**, 6 November, 1789–90.

Leopoldt, H., Corea, S. & Robinson, J.R. (1975) Hospital-based community psychiatric nursing in psychogeriatric care. *Nursing Mirror,* **141**, 18 December, 54–6.

Maggs, C.J. (1978) Towards a social history of nursing. *Nursing Times Occasional Papers* I and II, **74** (14), 18 May and **74** (15), 25 May.

Marks, I.M., Hallam, R.S., Connolly, J. & Philpott, R. (1977) *Nursing in Behavioural Psychotherapy.* Royal College of Nursing, London.

Marks, I.M., Hallam, R.S. & Philpott, R. (1976) Behavioural nurse therapists? The implications. *Nursing Times Occasional Paper,* **72** (19), 69–71.

Martin, R. (1975) *Developing an extended nursing role. The clinical nurse specialist/consultant in relation to neurosurgery.* Unpublished report.

McPhail, A. (1978) From head nurse to nurse manager. *The Canadian Nurse,* January, 32–9.

Merrison Report (1975) *Committee of Inquiry into the Regulation of the Medical Profession.* HMSO, London.

Merrison Report (1979) *Royal Commission on the National Health Service.* HMSO, London.

Millar, E.C. (1976) Letter on nurse specialists. *Nursing Times,* **72**, 16 December, 1970.

Miller, D.S. & Backett, E.M. (1980) A new member of the team? Extending the role of the nurse in British primary care. *Lancet,* 16 August, No. 8190, Vol. **2**, 358–61.

Millington, C. (1976) Clinical nurse consultant in anaesthetics. *Nursing Mirror,* **142** (20), 49–50.

MoH (1966) *Report of the Committee on Senior Nursing Staff Structure.* Chairman, Brian Salmon. HMSO, London.

Morgans, K.A. (1975) *Why a nurse for stoma care?* 1975 Stoma Care Symposium, ed. R.G. Richardson. Abbott Laboratories Ltd 1976, Queenborough, Kent.

National Association for Mental Health (1977) Another role for nurses! *Nursing Times*, **73**, 14 July, 1060.

National League for Nursing (1952) Nursing Education Division. *Report of the Work Conference on Graduate Nurse Education*. A conference of schools offering programs leading to a degree for graduate nurses, held at University of Chicago, 8–11 September. The League, New York (mincographed).

NLNE (1943) *Statement of Intent*. National League for Nursing Education, Washington DC.

Newton, J., Barnes, G., Cameron, J., Goldman, P. & Elias, J. (1976) Nurse specialists in family planning. *British Medical Journal*, **1**, 950–2.

Newton, M.P., Reed, C. & Close, A. (1977) Nurse specialist work in family planning. *Midwives Chronicle and Nursing Notes*, December, 290–1.

Nursing Mirror (1977) Editorial. *Nursing Mirror*, **145** (13).

Nursing Mirror (1976) Editorial. *Nursing Mirror*, **143** (5), 33.

Nursing Times (1976) Clinical nurse consulted? Editorial. *Nursing Times*, **72** (46).

O'Connor, V. (1971) New clinical specialist – a growing breed. *Nursing Times*, **67** (41), 1276–9.

Osborne, S. (1978) The role of the specialist in the breast unit. *Nursing Times*, **74** (29), 1201–2.

Parker, M. (1976) Clinical nurse consultant in infection control. *Nursing Mirror*, **142** (20), 51–3.

Parkinson, M.W. (1977) The role of the area nurse: child health. *Nursing Times*, **73** (43), 1684–5.

Peplau, H. (1965) Specialisation in professional nursing. Reprinted from *Nursing Science*, August 1965, 268–98. In: *The Clinical Nurse Specialist: Interpretations*, ed. J.P. Riehl & J.W. McVay, 1973, Appleton Century Crofts, New York.

Peplau, H. (1978) Psychiatric nursing: role of nurses and psychiatric nurses. *International Nursing Review*, **25** (2), 218.

Pohl, M. (1965) Teaching activities of the nursing practitioner. *Nursing Research*, **14** (1), 11, 719–21.

Reiter, F. (1966) Nurse clinician. *American Journal of Nursing*, **66** (2), 274–80.

Rigby, C. (1978) Community liaison. *Nursing Times*, **74** (30), 1246.

Robinson, L. (1974) *Liaison Nursing: Psychological Approach to Patient Care*. P.A. Davis Co., Philadelphia.

Rogers, C.G. (1973) As guides to clinical nursing specialisation. *Journal of Nursing Education*, November, 2–6.

RCN (1975) *New horizons in clinical nursing*. Report of a seminar held at Leeds Castle, Kent, 14–17 October. Royal College of Nursing, London.

RCN (1977) Evidence to the Royal Commission on the NHS, March 1977. Royal College of Nursing, London.

Saunders, B. (1976) Clinical nurse consultant in stoma care. *Nursing Mirror*, **142** (20), 54–8.

Simms, L.L. (1966) The clinical nursing specialist: an approach to nursing practice in the hospital. *Journal of the American Medical Association*, **198** (6), 207–9.

Smoyak, S.A. (1976) Specialisation in nursing: from then to now. *Nursing Outlook*, **24** (11), 676–81.

Stephens, D.S.B. & Boaler, J. (1977) The nurse's role in immediate postoperative care. *Nursing Mirror*, **145** (13), 20–23.

Tiffany, R. (1976) Department of Nursing Studies, Royal Marsden Hospital Annual Report. (Reference to the JBCNS course at the Royal Marsden Hospital and the concept of the clinical specialist.) *Nursing Mirror*, **141**, 14 August, 66–8.

Wald, F. & Leonard, R. (1964) Towards a development of nursing practice theory. *Nursing Research*, **13** (309).

Weller, B.F. (1971) A plea for a clinical specialty. *Nursing Times*, **67** (18), 552–3.

Whyte, B. (1977) Constant change is here to stay. *Nursing Mirror*, **144** (22), 17–18.

Wilson-Barnett, J. (1976) Reflections on progress. *Nursing Times*, **72** (25), 962.

Winder, E. (1977) One organ medicine. *British Medical Journal*, No. 6102, Vol. **2**, 1585–6.

Yokes, J.A. (1966) The clinical specialist in cardiovascular nursing. *American Journal of Nursing*, December, 2667–70.

Chapter 2

Clinical Specialists in Nursing in the UK: 1980s to the Present Day

George Castledine

Introduction

In the early 1980s the first piece of UK research on nurse specialists was carried out. Its purpose was to identify clinical nurse specialists in England and Wales, as defined by themselves and area health authorities. The study also aimed to compare their present development with that of clinical nurse specialists in other countries, particularly the USA (Castledine, 1982).

The study identified 353 perceived clinical nurse specialists in England and Wales, of which 49 were self-defined. Only 8% of the population came significantly near to fulfilling the role of a clinical nurse specialist. The job content of the potential clinical nurse specialists was diverse. None fulfilled all the essential characteristics of the clinical nurse specialist. The most common areas where they failed to do this were:

(1) The academic nursing education required for the role – only two of the 353 nurses held an MSc in clinical nursing.
(2) The amount and type of nursing research they were involved in was extremely limited.
(3) Published results of specialist work or articles relating to the specialty were rare.
(4) The nurses were often tied to the traditional barriers of a ward or service area and had to conform to line authority.
(5) Nursing process was often talked about but there was little evidence of its use in clinical practice.
(6) Though described as freelance practitioners and consultants who determined when and where their services were needed, it was not clear how and to whom they were accountable for their practice.

The development and progress of clinical nurse specialists in England and Wales in the early 1980s, compared with that in other countries such as the USA, was still confined to the medical profession's model of areas for specialization. Peplau's identification in 1965 of ten possible categories for specialization in nursing was a major step towards showing the fragmentation and diversity of opinion about such a development in the USA. Castledine's (1982) research supported Peplau's findings in relation to developments in England and Wales some 16 years later.

In outlining the development and progress of clinical nurse specialists in England and Wales, compared with that in other countries, Peplau (1965), in her historical perspective of specialization in America, pointed out that:

'Initially, the patterning of specialization is determined by avant garde workers in the particular field who see or sense a great need to move – in depth – in a particular direction. With regard to the profession of nursing, at first particular nurses move in a direction that interests them or towards which they have an immediate opportunity.'

It would appear from Castledine's (1982) research that this is exactly what has happened in England and Wales. Nurses have followed an interest which has taken them into a position of becoming a specialist and consultant on certain nursing matters. The majority of these nurses have followed this path at the expense of further post-registration and graduate education in clinical nursing. As Peplau (1965) pointed out, 'Over a period of time some of these directions survive and some of them don't.' In the UK their survival has been due, it would seem, to a group of very dedicated and enthusiastic specialist nurses.

The research in 1982 indicated that although many senior nurse managers recognized the existence of an expert specialist nurse they had done very little to encourage and support their development. For example, it was only after prolonged years in a certain post that some of the specialist nurses were promoted to a higher salary grade. Senior nursing managers claim that the reason for this poor recognition is not entirely their fault because they have been restricted by the rigid hierarchical nursing structure and the many changes that have taken place in nursing. A typical response by a nurse manager was:

'What else can I do? The nurse specialist does not fit very easily into the present nursing structure; she is not a manager so I could not justify her appointment at a higher level than a ward sister.'

It would also seem that it is not only fitting the nurse specialist into the present nursing structure which causes problems, but understanding the function of the role. The majority of the job descriptions which Castledine (1982) examined were vague and lacked any insight into what was actually happening in practice. When questioned about the vagueness and generality of such job descriptions, a typical nurse manager's response was:

'What else can I state about the job; I am not sure myself exactly what this nurse does. She gets on very well with the doctors, and the patients think she is marvellous.'

It was interesting to note the support given by the medical staff and perhaps this was one of the factors which determined the survival of a specialist nursing post. Castledine (1982) noted that where a particular specialist nurse was held in high esteem by all health care workers, the doctors played a significant role in backing up the nurse. From the research there were other 'pioneer' potential clinical nurse specialists whose success relied on their own initiative and hard work. Such nurses lacked the back-up experienced by many of the respondents who scored so highly on the questionnaire. There is a need, it would seem, for groups of nurses to get together and support new innovations. Peplau (1965) suggested that:

'Masses of nurses must become aware of individual efforts, learn enough about them to debate their merits, and give them sufficient support so that creative and constructive innovations can continuously be flowing into professional nursing.'

One significant finding by Peplau, and very applicable to Castledine's (1982) work, was her identification of ten specialty practice areas and two particular models used in other professional fields where clinical specialization in nursing was developing. From the analysis carried out by Castledine it would seem that the same situation existed in clinical specialization in nursing in England and Wales, well over a decade later.

Two particular models quoted by Peplau are also directions which specialization in this country could have followed. Social work at first followed and then discarded the medical model. 'Casework' with individual clients became more important, followed by 'group work' and 'community work'. Nursing in the UK is also focusing on or trying to encourage a similar pattern to this (i.e. the one-to-one relationship using the nursing process approach).

The second model described by Peplau, and which Castledine believed was developing in the UK, was that of 'clinical co-ordinator'. Nurses and doctors tend to use the phrases 'patient care' and 'nursing care' as if they were synonymous, which they are not. For example, in a geriatric health care team there may be several different specialist workers caring for the same patient. One nurse could not only co-ordinate the care given by the community and hospital nurses to the patient but could also act as overall co-ordinator of all the other services including the medical treatment. Therefore as patient care becomes more complex, demanding more experts, some nurses are functioning as the main co-ordinators of the patients' health care.

Reiter (1966), who was one of the first proponents of the clinical nurse as an expert practitioner, has maintained that the term 'clinical nurse specialist' is a generic and not a functional title:

> 'The practice of the clinical nurse specialist encompasses all the dimensions on which patient care is built.'

Based on this premise, the title 'clinical nurse specialist' signified a degree of knowledge and competence that a nurse had acquired in clinical practice; it did not signify a specific job or position he/she might hold in an employing authority. A significant number of senior nurse managers felt that this was true of many of the nurses which they had proposed for Castledine's research in 1982. In some situations they had backed up this belief by promoting the nurse, but had encouraged them to continue their present work without any additional responsibilities. There is no doubt that the way the nurse specialists in Castledine's research used their knowledge and skills in actual nursing care, and the extent to which they assumed specific roles – such as teacher, consultant, co-ordinator, researcher and so forth – varied according to the setting in which they practised.

Some of the other variables which may affect the nurse specialist role are the kinds of nursing problems with which the specialist deals. For example, a health education nurse was dealing with adolescent potential health problems whereas another nurse specializing with adolescent patients was dealing with actual health problems and the effects of a disease. There were stoma nurses who not only dealt with problems relating to the patient's stoma but had specialized further and were dealing with sexual problems. Castledine's research found out that very few specialists could produce written criteria based on a specific model of nursing. In the main, therefore, many of the problems which were highlighted related to the patients' medical treatment and physical problems.

There was no doubt from the observations which Castledine made at the time that:

(1) The majority of clinical nurse specialists were involved in direct nursing with patients.
(2) Patient accountability varied.
(3) Although many specialist nurses lacked a degree in nursing, their knowledge and expertise was sought after, and many of them had developed a body of nursing knowledge about their specialty which should have been further published and used. Unfortunately, many of the respondents felt that publishing was a low priority and, therefore, little of their work has been passed on in this way.
(4) Much of the research which these respondents were involved in was medically generated and oriented.

(5) Nurse specialists were very heavily committed to teaching, not only other nurses but paramedics, junior doctors and, of course, patients. It was significant that each specialist had developed some type of teaching programme and care plan for their patients. In many cases special booklets, written by the specialist nurse, had been printed for the patient.

(6) All the nurse specialists appeared to get on very well with other health care workers, especially when they were involved in discussions about a patient's future.

(7) There was great demand on the nurse specialist's time. Several of the nurse specialists were finding this pressure difficult to cope with and because they were working on their own, found themselves working very long hours.

(8) Time for writing articles, etc., about nursing care was extremely limited, especially during their officially specified working hours. This may have been one of the reasons why publishing came as a very low priority in their work.

(9) It would seem that at least some of the nurse specialists had a definite role of liaison between hospital and the community, thus ensuring continuity of nursing care.

The role of the nurse specialist

It is perhaps a fallacy to speak of the role of the clinical nurse specialist as though there were only one role and as though this one role had been clearly established. Christman (1965) criticized nurses in the USA for being too concerned with their role instead of being more concerned with the patient's nursing needs. It was not the intention of Castledine's 1982 research to stereotype an occupational role for the clinical nurse specialist. Therefore, an ideal job description was not attempted in those days. The number of different nurse specialists and the wide background from which they came prevented this.

Early specialization, however, in England and Wales more or less conformed to the medical profession's model of areas for specialization. Advanced preparation for nurses in these areas was very poor and usually took second place to educational preparation for nursing management and teaching. Nursing education, to a large extent, shared in perpetuating the notion that all nurses must be equipped to care for all kinds of patients in a variety of settings. There are indications from Castledine's 1982 research that one of the fundamental problems in nursing is that education and hospital nursing management, in particular, have failed to come to grips with the role of clinical nurse specialists. One of the effects of increasing technology and specialization in patient care is that the concept of general nursing is becoming more unrealistic and in some areas impossible.

How clinical nurse specialists operates within an institution or community depends very much on how a health authority wants to use them. From Castledine's 1982 research it would seem that to become such a nurse specialist, a nurse must have practised nursing, continue to practise and continue to evolve through practising nursing. The nurse's practice with patients must be deliberate, systematic, reflective, analytic, innovative and dynamic. Nurses are proving in many situations to be the model of expertise to beat traditional methods of nursing by stimulating and taking part in nursing research.

It would seem that the nurse's practice is enhanced when he or she is not assigned to a nursing unit but is free to follow patients wherever their requirements for nursing care may take them within the organization. In many situations it would seem that the nurse's practice should not be bound by the hospital walls but reach out to the patient at home in the community. At present, it is through clinical nurse specialists that clinical teaching and clinical nursing practice are being kept together.

There has been considerable discussion about which term – extended or expanded – should be used to describe the role of the clinical nurse specialist. Generally the term 'extended role' has been used to describe the nurse's professional acts which have moved into what was at one time a grey area between medical and nursing practice. Some nurses have rejected this term in favour of the term 'expanded role', arguing that the nurse has expanded his or her role in depth and scope of professional acts that are inherently nursing and not medical in nature. Abdellah *et al.* (1973) stated that:

> 'Although the clinical nurse specialist may practice with patients who manifest a rather narrow clinical problem, her practice has a broader frame of reference. For example, the nurse who cares for patients with ostomies might (hopefully she will) find that future medical science or surgical techniques are developed to eliminate the need for an ostomy. This same nurse would have no difficulty at all shifting her practice to patients with amputations, for example.'

In the UK, individual groups within the profession have struggled long and hard to define a clinical career structure in nursing. For many years, they have given a great deal of thought to issues such as how to describe clinical expertise and development and what title to give clinical developers. Despite much debate, many problems and difficulties remain.

A Department of Health (DoH, 1995) document highlighted the factors that influence career development for qualified practitioners, employers and educationalists and the diversity of career roles and opportunities available. In 1979, Friend set up a working group within the nursing division of the Department of Health to examine the available evidence and identify the main difficulties inhibiting the implementation of a clinical career structure for nursing (Friend, 1980). It was found that:

(1) Careers in clinical nursing should be soundly based on post-registration education and experience
(2) Some nurses were being appointed into senior clinical posts without the appropriate education and training
(3) The role of the then nursing officer was too removed from practice and there should be more clinically based senior nursing officers with wider responsibilities
(4) The appointment of an experienced clinical nurse to act as facilitator and leader should be considered
(5) There should be a 'single spine' nursing pay structure

Role extension/expansion in the 1990s
(The Scope of Professional Practice)

The role and functions undertaken by nurses, midwives and health visitors appear largely to have been guided by policy emanating from the Department of Health and the statutory bodies. In 1977 the Department of Health and Social Security issued guidance on the extended role of the nurse (DHSS, 1977), which Carlisle (1992) regarded as ludicrous. Certification of nurses to undertake specific skills was often granted by people not involved in the education process and only considered valid within the practitioner's speciality. Extended role functions were, therefore, widely viewed as stifling rather than enhancing practice.

The introduction of *The Scope of Professional Practice* by the United Kingdom Central Council (UKCC, 1992) replaced the guidance on extended roles and allowed the development and adaptation of roles to meet changing need. It emphasized the practitioner's professional accountability and placed decisions concerning competence in the hands of the individual. Moores (1992) proclaimed that the UKCC document presented an opportunity for individual practitioners to build and develop the interests of patient care 'in the round' while exercising full professional accountability. The document also replaced the term 'extended role' with 'expanded role'. Greenhalgh (1994) made the distinction between role extension and expansion by defining the former as acceptance of new tasks, frequently from other groups and most often involving technical skills. The skills acquired in role extension are a result of training rather than education, and nursing or paramedic education is not prerequisite. Role expansion on the other hand is defined as the decision to learn based on each practitioner's situation.

In addition to advances in medicine, the pressure for change in the practitioner's role has been influenced by comprehensive ideological change in the form of the National Health Service and Community Care Act 1990 and the creation of the internal market. These reforms have demanded an examination of the way in which health care is delivered and have focused attention on the roles and responsibilities of those professionals who deliver it. This is reflected clearly in the community where the blurring of roles is extending from health into social care. The pressure to deliver services on a need basis requires not only a more efficient use of health care personnel, but also one that is more effective in producing clear and positive patient/client outcomes. The Patient's Charter (DoH, 1991) acknowledged that both outcomes and consumer satisfaction could be improved by identifying key workers and proposed the introduction of the 'named' nurse. It is also clear from the *Health of the Nation* targets (DoH, 1992) that nurses, midwives and health visitors will play a vital role in reducing risk and promoting the health of their clients.

There is a further issue which has a significant effect in determining the role of practitioners and that is the reduction in junior doctors' hours (DoH, 1991). Regional task forces were established and charged with the responsibility of ensuring that targets for reducing junior doctors' hours were achieved. Greenhalgh (1994) identified a split in opinion among regions as to the extent of the nursing and midwifery contribution to this reduction, but the West Midlands regional task force suggested that 'nurse practitioner' could assist in the partial elimination of a medical tier. Ashcroft (1992) supported the idea of nurse/midwife substitution of particular medical technical tasks and argued that junior doctor rotation demanded a steep learning curve which resulted in less than optimum care, whereas nurses and midwives, experienced in their field, would remain competent through constant practice. Findings from Greenhalgh and Company (Greenhalgh, 1994) indicated that where nursing substitution occurred in six main activities such as cannulation, there was no statistical difference in quality between the doctors and nurses undertaking those activities.

Dowling *et al.* (1995) expressed the view that innovations in the division of labour required as rigorous evaluation as new surgical techniques and that there should be an identification and understanding of the essential and generalized features of new working practice. Dowling also argued that nursing substitution of a large proportion of medical duties is neither a cheap nor easy solution.

The essence of the ideological shift in health care and the effect on the practitioner's role is embodied in the Heathrow Debate (DoH, 1994). This discusses the influences for change and attempts to predict the role of nursing and midwifery in the future. A polarization of nursing is envisaged, where the split of primary and secondary care will produce very distinct practitioners. Demand and technological innovation will mean that there will be community health and illness prevention practitioners, together with long term, fundamental care roles and high dependency, acute and specialist hospital carers, whose function will be paramedic in orientation. However, consensus was reached regarding what is constant in nursing:

'The work of the nurse, whatever the setting, draws upon a tradition of caring, based around both skills and values.' (DoH, 1994)

Identified as part of this constant were six functions: co-ordinating; teaching carers, patients and professions; developing and maintaining programmes of care; technical expertise; concern for both the ill and well; and special responsibility for the frail and vulnerable. Agreement concerning the nature of nursing has always posed problems but unless consensus is reached and there is a clear definition of the nursing role, Denner (1995) argued, no one can say the direction nursing should go in the future. The specialization of roles and the diversity of their nature provides a clear rationale for placing accountability for practice in the hands of the individual.

More recently, with dramatic advances in medical technology, specialized intensive care units and surgical procedures and the need to reduce the number of hours worked by junior doctors, there has been a renewed interest in the possibilities for developing advanced nurse practitioners to relieve the stresses on medical staff and increase the nurses' responsibilities. Dowling *et al.* (1995) described the differences in role, satisfaction and effectiveness of nurses who had undertaken posts in which they were performing substantially house officer and senior house officer roles. They found that those posts where nurses were substituted for house officers for expediency were less successful practically and economically, while the post developed specifically to improve patient care, and which involved considerable planning and education of the post holder, increased personal job satisfaction and effectiveness of care.

The expansion of the practitioner's role was seen as a positive move by Moyse (1994) who viewed the production of the *Scope of Practice* guidelines as a means to facilitate the reduction in junior doctors' hours, but suggested that practitioners were using the opportunity to develop practice. Cohen (1995) felt that the Royal College of Nursing/British Medical Association had been keen to stress the opportunities for nursing and midwifery, but supported Dowling (1995) in identifying that role substitution is not a cheap option.

Through its work on the code of conduct and in particular *The Scope of Professional Practice* the UKCC (1992) has opened the door to further expansion and development in clinical nursing practice. Since its publication and wide distribution in 1992, *The Scope of Professional Practice* has been acknowledged in many quarters as a bold and imaginative response to the needs of patients and clients for innovative approaches to care. In addition it has addressed the needs of practitioners for greater satisfaction from their professional practice. It implies that the practitioner has the autonomy and accountability to develop and practice skills within their profession, and suggests the blurring of boundaries between professions and disciplines as to role functions.

Professional practice is defined as practice which is sensitive, relevant and responsive to the needs of individual patients and clients and has the capacity to adjust, where and when appropriate, to changing circumstances (UKCC, 1992). There are six principles laid out for adjusting the scope of practice:

(1)   The interests and needs of the patient must be paramount
(2)   Nurses must improve their levels of skill and knowledge before taking on any new roles
(3)   Nurses must be aware of themselves and their duty to improve and develop
(4)   Nurses must be aware of the extent of their skills and knowledge and not compromise or fragment existing practice
(5)   In all such developments the nurse will be held personally accountable
(6)   When taking on new role developments the nurse must avoid any inappropriate delegation to other health care personnel.

Within pre-registration education and practice, the nurse will be prepared to develop competence to practice. As education and development must be proved as a continuous process throughout the career span of a practitioner, it is obvious that some progression of these skills will develop at different levels and at different stages for individuals. Presently there are various educational routes to facilitate these developments.

Throughout the UK there have been several initiatives in response to the UKCC's *Scope of Professional Practice* (Touche Ross & Co, 1994). The Department of Health is committed to developments which improve the contribution made to health gains and health care by nurses and to the need to improve the living and working conditions, clinical experiences and training of junior doctors (Greenhalgh, 1994).

Confusion and abuse of titles and roles

Despite the efforts of the UKCC to encourage the development of nursing specialists and in particular a clinical career structure for nurses following its Post Registration Education and Practice (PREP) recommendations, other developments and influences both from within the UK and in particular from North America, have hampered and confused the progress of clarifying what it is nurses should be specializing in. In particular, the following four factors have played a significant part:

(1) Physicians' assistants in North America
(2) Nurse practitioners/nurse clinicians in North America
(3) The UK nurse practitioners movement
(4) Physicians' assistants in the UK.

These are discussed in turn here.

Physicians' assistants in North America

In autumn 1970 in California, a bill (A62109) was introduced which directed the Board of Medical Examiners to establish a new category of health care personnel called physicians' assistants. Steeg (1975) pointed out that this law was to have a great effect on the development of the concept of physicians' assistants throughout the USA. The origins of the movement were founded in the belief:

> 'that there was a huge shortage of health care personnel – specifically physicians and nurses and a flood of returning veterans who had acquired technical skills under military–medical auspices. What more logical solution than to hive these well trained "medics" to work in civilian settings.' (Steeg, 1975)

The relevance of physicians' assistants to this study was supported by Bullough's (1975) comments about nurses expanding their scope of practice to take on new responsibilities:

> 'For a time it looked as if this would not be possible because of psychological and legal barriers created by past subordination and by the nurses' own response to that subordination. In fact, the impetus for the expanding role is largely due to forces outside nursing.'

It would seem that apart from the shortages of physicians, it was the trend towards specialization in medicine which had also played its part in creating a gap in the health care delivery system. This 'gap', as Bullough (1975) saw it, had to be filled by someone and the vital question was whether nursing should take on this work or if a new type of health worker should be developed. In 1975, in the USA, it would seem that young men who had been working in the armed services as medical assistants would be the ideal people to fit this role; however, there were some disadvantages to the physicians' assistants approach. The supply of discharged men was limited and their training was at first restricted to about ten weeks' experience. More recently this situation has significantly changed and three year degree programmes have been developed for aspiring physicians' assistants.

The introduction of physicians' assistants in other countries, particularly China and the USSR, appeared to have been fairly successful as documented by Sidel and Sidel (1973) and Field (1972). The crux of the matter lay in the need for basic changes in the system of finance in patterns of medical practice, and in the content of medical education.

The transfer of medical functions and responsibilities from physicians to nurses extends back to the time when nurses were first entrusted with using medical instruments, such as a thermometer, in their nursing care of patients; however, in reality it represents a quantum leap and threatens the fundamental principles on which the practice of nursing was established (Farmer, 1995). To move professionally educated nurses from nursing roles so that they can function at a lower level in the field of medicine is an unbelievable human and intellectual waste and denies patients the benefits of nursing care provided by experts.

The idea of following the medical model is very attractive to those nurses who do not think that nursing has a destiny of its own or who believe that their identity and status will not be enhanced if they follow a nursing model. Also, some nurses may feel that the medical model offers them greater challenges and responsibilities. However, many are now realizing that nurses can never really have a lone identity, freedom and autonomy using the medical model.

The medical model focuses on signs, symptoms, pathology, prognosis and the course of the disease. This disease-oriented approach not only emphasizes the structure and functions of the body rather than the total person, but also has influenced the development of specialization in the medical profession. There is a danger that we may follow this medical approach in nursing and have nurse specialists roles based on certain organs, illnesses or functions of the body.

Specialization in nursing is usually seen as a mark of advancement and progress, but we have to be certain that it is the nursing elements that are being developed and not medical functions as carried out by nurses.

Nurse practitioners in North America

The American Nurses' Association (ANA, 1976) defined the nurse practitioner as:

'having advanced skills in the assessment of the physical and psychosocial health-illness status of individuals, families or groups in a variety of settings.

They are prepared for these special skills by formal continuing education which adheres to the American Nurses' Association approved guidelines or in a baccalaureate nursing programme.'

The term 'nurse practitioner' appears to have originated in 1965 with the establishment of the paediatric nurse practitioner programme at the University of Colorado by Henry Silver and Loretta Ford. The shortages of medical manpower and increased medical specialization referred to above resulted in an upsurge of interest in the nurse practitioner movement.

It was not until later, however, that research data was available with regard to this development in nursing. The most important first longitudinal study of nurse practitioners was carried out by Harry Sultz at the State University of New York at Buffalo from 1973 onwards (Sultz, 1976): the study of nurse practitioner training programmes and their students, and phase 2 based on questionnaires sent to graduates of the nurse practitioner programmes to elicit data on job choice, employability and satisfaction. The results of this study showed that 57.4% of nurse practitioners were employed by physicians and 80.5% were supervised directly by a physician.

One interesting finding was that only about half the nurse graduates in this role used the title 'nurse practitioner'. The rest used such titles as 'nurse associate', 'nurse clinician', 'clinical nurse specialist', or 'nurse midwife'. Finally, barriers to the development of the nurse practitioner role were seen as arising from a variety of sources, legal barriers being the most frequently cited and resistance from other health care providers coming a close second. Very few studies have evaluated the nurse practitioner role, probably because it would require a considerable length of time to study the relationship between care provided by nurse practitioners and client outcomes. As Levine (1977) pointed out, 'measuring "quality" of care is difficult. Most evaluations of practitioners are anecdotal and appraise nursing process rather than client outcomes.'

Cohen and others at the Yale University School of Medicine (Cohen *et al.*, 1974) carried out an extensive review of evaluating nurse practitioners; they found that health practitioners in general (a term embracing nurse practitioners and physicians' assistants) had:

(1) Saved the physician time
(2) Been profitable to some employers
(3) Provided continuity of care where care had obviously been fragmented
(4) Been accepted by consumers
(5) Provided a performance level that compares favourably to physicians, as judged by standards developed within practice settings.

Ostergaard *et al.* (1975) referred to physicians' assistants and nurse practitioners as 'women's health-care specialists (WHCS)'. Although these were limited to the field of obstetrics and gynaecology, they felt that there were many advantages to the physician who employed such a person, such as relieving the physician of routine screening for disease, and helping in the insertion of intrauterine devices. A similar situation was described by Newton *et al.* (1976). They described the work of nursing in dispensing oral contraceptives, inserting intrauterine devices and diagnosing side effects in an experimental clinic run by nurse specialists in family planning at King's College Hospital, London. Critics of using nurses in family planning have often emphasized the inability of the nurse specialist to diagnose side effects and fit devices; however, Newton supported the use of a nurse in this work by illustrating the success of such a project with 778 patients seen by specialist nurses in their first year. A more critical question, therefore, is how such a role may further the cause of nursing as an independent and unique profession.

Perhaps Newton and his colleagues (1976) would answer this by pointing out 'the importance of a female attendant', that 'we think that the patient discusses her particular problems better with a nurse than with a doctor', and 'the enthusiasm shown by the nurse specialists for this type of work', combined and brought with it something very special to the caring relationship with the patient and the physician.

In the debate of care versus cure, care traditionally has been the domain of nursing and cure the domain of medicine. Linn (1974) pointed out from her study of a family nurse practitioner programme that nurses who were educated for extended roles did not abandon nursing values and orientation. Using an attitude survey and response categorization technique, Linn (1974) found that medical views were cure-oriented and nursing views care-oriented, and that although in their training nurse practitioners were taught medical skills, concepts and procedures, they still did not 'adopt traditional medical views'.

Linn concluded her study by stating:

'At least in terms of attitudes toward patient care and the system in which it occurs, this study seems to show that nurse practitioners represent a fusion of values from nursing and medicine.'

A controlled study of the effectiveness of paediatric nurse practitioners with pre-school children carried out by Burnip *et al.* (1976) supported their competence, acceptance by patients' families and cost effectiveness. The National Commission for Manpower Policy (1976) concluded that:

'the greater acceptance of the role of physician extenders (meaning nurse practitioners and physician assistants) and the greater recognition of the increase in system efficiency that can result from this new division of labour comes at the very moment when the supply of physicians is increasing dramatically. To some degree, therefore, the relative need for physician extenders will decline.'

Recent literature from North America suggests this decline has not happened. It would seem, however, that this study assumes that the only reason for the existence of nurse practitioners is to do the tasks relegated by physicians, and that as the shortage of physicians ends there will no longer be any need for such people. Levine (1977) points out, however, that this view may be very short sighted as:

'many studies, although lacking in acceptable research design and inconclusive in results, strongly suggest that the nurse practitioner role is efficient, effective and produces high quality outcomes. This, plus an easing of legal barriers and the possibility of direct reimbursement for services, appears to favour an expansion in the use of nurse practitioners in the future.'

Nurse clinicians in North America

The American Nurses' Association (ANA, 1976) defined the nurse clinician as:

'having well-developed competencies in utilizing a broad range of cues. These cues are used for prescribing and implementing both direct and indirect nursing care and for articulating nursing therapies with other planned therapies. Nurse clinicians demonstrate expertise in nursing practice and ensure on-going development of expertise through clinical experience and continuing education. Generally minimal preparation for this role is the baccalaureate degree.'

In 1976, however, the American Nurses' Association decided to drop the term clinician as a separate entity and integrate this title with that of nurse practitioner:

'since consistent and significant differences in education, practice or place of practice could not be identified, the term practitioner/clinician be used and the description of practice apply to both roles.' (ANA, 1976)

The UK nurse practitioner movement

The use of the term 'nurse practitioner' to refer to nurses who have taken on new functions specifically related to medical knowledge and medical tasks is an abuse of the term. There is no universally accepted definition of a nurse practitioner (Castledine, 1995); indeed, some nurses have used it in its literal sense to apply to any nurse, whatever their discipline or field of nursing. The Royal College of Nursing has promoted the use of the term to refer to a special nurse in the community who helps a GP by assessing certain groups of patients and performing medical tasks and health promotion activities.

Gaze (1985) reported the difficulties faced by one of the first nurse practitioners in the UK when she tried to take on a more medical role by prescribing drugs for patients. Stilwell (1985), however, in evaluating the role of the nurse practitioner, highlighted the nursing aspects of the role and likened her work to that of nurse practitioners in Canada and the USA. The nurse practitioner movement has continued to develop in the UK since Stilwell's early work, and it is now recognized as equivalent to specialist nursing and the clinical nurse specialist.

The content and function of role are important issues for the individual practising as a nurse practitioner. There should be a clearer distinction between nurses who are primarily focusing on medicine, and nurse practitioners who are integrating medicine into their primary nursing role. Nursing should never be seen as second-class medicine and nurses should be proud to use the term 'nursing' in any description of their role.

The term nurse practitioner has also been used in hospital settings. For example, the Royal College of Nursing's Accident and Emergency Association defines the emergency nurse practitioner as:

'An A&E nurse who has a sound nursing practice base in all aspects of A&E nursing with formal post-basic education in holistic assessment, physical diagnosis, prescription of treatment and promotion of health.' (Jones, 1994)

Jones (1994) rightly pointed out that the concept of a nurse seeing patients, and treating and discharging them without reference to a doctor, is not new. Many minor casualty units, usually in rural areas, have provided this type of service for a number of years.

The title 'night nurse practitioner' is another example of the use of the term. Morley (1992) suggested potential areas of practice for night nurse practitioners, e.g. resiting venous cannulae, administering intravenous medications, carrying out electrocardiograms, certification of expected deaths, and male catheterization. The argument in favour of continuing these posts is that they save medical time and improve continuity of patient care.

However, nurses who move into this paramedical field may be placing their nursing careers at risk by ending up in a 'career cul-de-sac', i.e. they may find themselves ostracized from the mainstream of nursing development and career opportunity. To avoid this and prevent isolation, these nurses should be seeking to clarify which aspects of their work require medical judgments and which require nursing judgments. All nurses regularly make rapid and sound decisions about whether to make clinical judgments in the medical domain or to diagnose in the nursing domain (Hannah *et al.*, 1987). The extent to which they focus on nursing probably determines whether their role is biased towards medicine or nursing.

Physicians' assistants in the UK

There are a small number of nurses working as technicians to surgeons in the UK. The most famous example is Susanne Holmes who worked in Oxford transferring and preparing veins for a cardiac surgeon. The most significant part of such a nurse's role is related to medicine and helping the physician or surgeon. Therefore, it is perhaps more appropriate to refer to these individuals as paramedical nurse practitioners and define them as:

> 'someone who is able to demonstrate the necessary knowledge and skill to supplement and support a physician or surgeon in his/her medical work. They will have acquired knowledge and skill in the medical field and be accountable to a doctor.' (Castledine, 1997a)

Examples of such nurses are physicians' and surgeons' assistants, nurse clinicians, technicians and some nurse practitioners who focus primarily on medicine in their role or who work as a GP's assistant.

The term 'paramedical' is used in its strictest sense, i.e. one who supplements the work of the medical profession. A possible alternative title could be a medical health care worker.

Collaboration and co-operation between doctors and nurses

Until recently, doctors and nurses have often, openly or otherwise, resisted the philosophy of collaboration and some doctors still have difficulty in accepting nurses as equals in the health care team.

There is now considerable evidence, for example Hanna (1996), to show that nurses are much better than their medical colleagues at patient consultation and giving health advice. At the National Association of GP Co-operatives' annual conference in Warwick, Castledine (1997b) reported that the predominant questions asked by doctors were: 'Are nurses up to this?'; 'Will they be as good as me?'; and 'In what way can I use my nurses to save time and money?'. Few doctors were keen to experiment with an independent nurse practitioner because of the associated legal and accountability issues, or so they claimed. However, not surprisingly, many were willing to use nurses for certain functional medical tasks and felt that they could easily train nurses to do what they wanted them to do.

Until recently, medicine has been perceived as a vocation which borders on the divine. In the past, this link was thought of as spiritual; today, however, the divine element is associated with the mysteries of science and technology. Being a doctor is an awesome responsibility but it generates many unrealistic expectations and prejudices.

In the USA, Jacobsen and Jacobsen (1994) reported that 50% of all patients had, at one time or another, stopped seeing their doctor because they were dissatisfied with him/her. In the UK, the public is becoming more uneasy about the way in which doctors behave, i.e. not giving them enough information. It is not surprising, therefore, that the medical profession is perceived as being a predominantly paternalistic clan or fraternity that is bound by internal solidarity to protect its erring members from public scrutiny or punitive action. In medical complaint cases, many nurses have found to their cost that doctors' loyalties lie first with their colleagues and then with their patients or nursing staff.

Doctors have power, but power corrupts. The way in which doctors often see the role of the nurse demonstrates not only their arrogance but also their ignorance of what nurses are achieving. The problem is that nurses themselves do not agree over what nursing is and the differences between the medical and nursing domains. Nurses allow themselves to be deflected away from the real issues of nursing, e.g. looking at their role merely as an institutional employee or as a substitute for other disciplines. The definition and theory of nursing have been sidetracked by issues such as what tasks doctors are able to delegate to nurses.

Although some doctors and employers talk about interdisciplinary care and collaboration, these may deflate the potential power of nursing. Nurses will continue to be confused about their specialist and advanced role if they forget where their core knowledge and competencies emanate from and become too preoccupied with mimicking medicine.

References

Abdellah, F.G., Belland, I.L., Martin, A. & Matheney, R.V. (1973) *New Directions in Patient Centered Nursing*. Macmillan, New York.

ANA (1976) *The Scope of Nursing Practice*. Document May 1976, chaired by I.G. Mauksch. American Nurses' Association.

Ashcroft, J. (1992) Rising to the challenge. *Nursing Times*, **88** (37), 30.

Bullough, B. (1975) Barriers to the nurse practitioner movement: problems of women in a woman's field. *International Journal of Health Services*, **5** (2), 225–33.

Burnip, R., Erickson, R., Barr, G.D., Shinefield, H. & Schoen, E.J. (1976) Well-child care by paediatric nurse practitioners in a large group practice. *American Journal Dis. Child*, **130**, Jan, 51–5.

Carnevali, D. & Little, D. (1967) Nurse specialist effect on tuberculosis. *Nursing Research*, **16** (4), 321–6.

Castledine, G. (1995) Will the nurse practitioner be a mini doctor or a maxi nurse? *British Journal of Nursing*, **4** (16), 938–9.

Castledine, G. (1982) *The role and function of clinical nurse specialists in England and Wales*. Unpublished MSc dissertation. University of Manchester.

Castledine, G. (1997a) Framework for a clinical career structure in nursing. *British Journal of Nursing*, **6** (5), 264–71.

Castledine, G. (1997b) Nurses must stop themselves being used by doctors. *British Journal of Nursing*, **6** (4), 234.

Christman, L. (1965) The influence of specialisation on the nursing profession. *Nursing Science*, **3** (6), 446–53.

Cohen, E.D. *et al.* (1974) *An Evaluation of Policy Related Research on New and Expanded Roles of Health Workers*, No. APR 73-07904A02, New Haven, Office of Regional Activities and Continuing Education, Yale University School of Medicine.

Cohen, P. (1995) Mixed feelings. *Nursing Times*, **89** (19), 25.

Denner, S. (1995) Extending professional practice: benefits and pitfalls. *Nursing Times*, **91** (14), 27–31.

DoH (1995) *Career Pathways: Nursing, Midwifery and Health Visiting*. HMSO, London.

DoH (1991) *The Patients Charter*. HMSO, London.

DoH (1992) *The Health of the Nation: A Strategy for Health in England*. HMSO, London.

DoH (1994) *The Challenges for Nursing and Midwifery in the 21st Century* (The Heathrow Debate). Department of Health, London.

DHSS (1977) *The Extending Role of the Clinical Nurse*. HC (77) 22, June 1977. HMSO, London.

Dowling, S., Barret, S. & West, R. (1995) With nurse practitioners, who needs house officers? *British Medical Journal*, **311**, 29 July, 309–13.

Farmer, E. (1995) Medicine and nursing: a marriage for the 21st century. *British Journal of Nursing*, **4** (14), 793–4.

Field, M.G. (1972) Comment. *Bulletin of The New York Academy of Medicine*, **48**, 83.

Friend, P. (1980) Careers in clinical nursing. Unpublished paper. Nursing Division, Department of Health, London.

Gaze, H. (1985) Out in the cold, nurse practitioners (news focus). *Nursing Times*, **81** (11), 13.

Greenhalgh (1994) *The Interface Between Junior Doctors and Nurses: A Research Study for the Department of Health*. Greenhalgh and Co, Macclesfield.

Hanna, D.L. (1996) Primary care. In: *Advanced Nursing Practice* (eds Hamric, A.B., Spross, J.A. & Hanson, C.M.), 337–50. W.B. Saunders, Philadelphia.

Hannah, K.J., Reimer, M., Mills, W.C. & Letournean, S.L. (1987) *Clinical Judgement and Decision Making: The Future with Nursing Diagnosis*. John Wiley & Sons, Toronto, Canada.

Jacobsen, D. & Jacobsen, E.D. (1994) *Doctors are Gods*. Thunder Mouth Press, New York.

Jones, G. (1994) Accident and emergency and the emergency nurse practitioner. In: *Expanding the Role of the Nurse* (eds Hunt, G. & Wainwright, P.), 162–80, Blackwell Science, Oxford.

Levine, E. (1977) What do we know about nurse practitioners? *American Journal of Nursing*, **40**, 1799–1803.

Linn, L.S. (1974) Care vs cure. How the nurse practitioner views the patient. *Nursing Outlook*, **22** (10), 641–4.

Moores, Y. (1992) Setting new boundaries. *Nursing Times*, **88** (37), 29.

Morley, B. (1992) Role of the night nurse practitioner. *British Journal of Nursing*, **1** (14), 719–21.

Moyse, G. (1994) No shuffling on new deal. *Nursing Management*, **1** (7), 27–8.

National Commission for Manpower Policy (1976) *Report of the National Advisory Commission on Health Manpower*, Vol. II. US Government Printing Office, Washington DC.

Newton, J., Barnes, G., Cameron, J., Goldman, P. & Elias, J. (1976) Nurse specialists in family planning. *British Medical Journal*, **1**, 950–2.

Ostergaard, D.R., Gunning, J.E. & Marshall, J.R. (1975) Training and function of a women's health care specialist, a physician's assistant, or nurse practitioner in obstetrics and gynaecology. *American Journal of Obstetrics and Gynecology*, **121** (8), 1029–37.

Peplau, H. (1965) Specialisation in professional nursing. Reprinted from *Nursing Science*, August 1965, 268–98. In: *The Clinical Nurse Specialist: Interpretations* (eds J.P. Riehl & J.W. McVay), 1973, Appleton Century Crofts, New York.

Reiter, F. (1966) Nurse clinician. *American Journal of Nursing*, **66** (2), 274–80.

Sidel, V.W. & Sidel, R. (1973) *Serve the People*, pp. 33, 41, 196. Jacobsen, New York.

Steeg, D.P.V. (1975) Development of physicians' assistants and nurse practitioners in California. *Bulletin of the New York Academy of Medicine*, **51** (2), 286–94.

Stilwell, B. (1985) Setting the scene: the nurse practitioner. *Nursing Mirror*, **160** (15), 15–16.

Sultz, H.A. (1976) *Longitudinal Study of Nurse Practitioners*. No. (HRA) 76-43, US Department of Health, Education and Welfare, Washington DC.

Touche & Ross & Co. (1994) *Evaluation of Nurse Practitioner Pilot Projects*. NHS Executive, South Thames, London.

UKCC (1992) *The Scope of Professional Practice*. UKCC, London.

Further reading

American Nurses Association (1995) Nursing's Social Policy Statement. ANA, Washington.

Ayers, R. (1971) *The Clinical Nurse Specialist – An Experiment in Role Effectiveness and Role Development*. Durato, California: City of Hope National Medical Center.

Berlinger, M.R. (1969) The preparation and roles of the clinical specialist at the master's level. Reprinted paper in *The Clinical Nurse Specialist: Interpretations* (eds J.P. Riehl & J.W. McVay), 1973, Appleton Century Crofts, New York.

Bicknell, W.J., Walsh, D.C. & Tanner, M.M. (1974) Substantial or decorative? Physicians' assistants and nurse practitioners in the USA. *Lancet*, **2**, 23 November, 1241–4.

British Association for Specialists in Clinical Nursing (1975) Letter describing the group's aims. *Nursing Mirror*, **143** (5), 43.

Brooks, C. (1976) Implementation of the role of the clinical nursing specialist in a health maintenance organisation. In: *Quality Patient Care and the Role of the Clinical Nursing Specialist* (ed. R. Rotkovitch). John Wiley & Sons, New York.

Brown, R. (1995) The politics of specialist/advanced practice: conflict or confusion? *British Journal of Nursing,* **4** (16), 944–8.

Burson, I.J. (1976) The clinical nursing specialist in paediatrics. In: *Quality Patient Care and the Role of the Clinical Nursing Specialist* (ed. R. Rotkovitch). John Wiley & Sons, New York.

Carlisle, D. (1992) Scope for extensions. *Nursing Times,* **88** (37), 26, 28.

Carlson, S. (1976) The department of nursing education in a health care agency and the role of the clinical nursing specialist. In: *Quality Patient Care and the Role of the Clinical Nursing Specialist* (ed. R. Rotkovitch). John Wiley & Sons, New York.

Cox, S. (1978) The introduction of nurse specialists. *Nursing Times,* **74** (27), 1125.

Dirschel, K.M. (1976) The conception, gestation and delivery of the clinical nursing specialist. In: *Quality Patient Care and the Role of the Clinical Nursing Specialist* (ed. R. Rotkovitch). John Wiley & Sons, New York.

Dumat, L.S. (1975) The role of the psychiatric clinical specialist in the haemodialysis unit. In: *The Clinical Nurse Specialist – A Symposium,* 4 April. Sigma Theta Tan National Honour Society of Nursing, Michigan.

Dunn, B.H. (1975) Role evolution of a clinical specialist/nurse practitioner in sub-specialty. In: *The Clinical Nurse Specialist – A Symposium,* 4 April. Sigma Theta Tan, Michigan.

Fieldman, H.R. (1976) The medical–surgical clinical nursing specialist. In: *Quality Patient Care and the Role of the Clinical Nursing Specialist* (ed. R. Rotkovitch). John Wiley & Sons, New York.

Georgopoulos, B.S. & Jackson, M.M. (1970) Nursing Kardex behaviour in an experimental study of patient units with and without clinical nurse specialists. *Nursing Research,* **19**, 196–218.

Georgopoulos, B.S. & Sana, J.M. (1971) Clinical nursing specialisation and intershift report behaviour. *American Journal of Nursing,* **71** (3), 538, 545.

Healy, P. (1996) Confusion reigns over nurse practitioners. *Nursing Standard,* **6** (11), 13.

Journal of Community Nursing (1981) *Danger: specialists at work.* Editorial. *Journal of Community Nursing,* **5** (1).

King's Fund (1978) *The New Health Practitioners in America – a Comparative Study,* by B.L. Reedy. King Edward's Hospital Fund for London.

MacPhail, J. (1971) Reasonable expectations for the nurse clinician. *Journal of Nursing Administration,* **1** (5), 16–18.

MacPhail, J. (1976) Reasonable expectations for the nurse clinician. In: *Clinical Specialists and Nurse Clinicians,* a reader by the *Journal of Nursing Administration,* Contemporary Pub., Massachusetts.

McGann, M.R. (1975) The clinical specialist: from hospital to clinic, to community. *Journal of Nursing Administration,* March/April. Reprinted in *Clinical Specialists and Nurse Clinicians, Journal of Nursing Administration* special reader, 1976, Contemporary Pub., Massachusetts.

McGee, P., Castledine, G. & Brown, R. (1996) A survey of specialist and advanced nursing practice in England. *British Journal of Nursing,* **5** (11), 682–6.

Millar, E.C. (1977) Nurse therapy in general practice. *Nursing Mirror,* **144**, 12 May, 47, 50.

Muschallo, J. (1976) The clinical nursing specialist and nursing specialist and nursing care co-ordinator in obstetrics. In: *Quality Patient Care and the Role of the Clinical Nursing Specialist* (ed. R. Rotkovitch). John Wiley & Sons, New York.

National League for Nursing (1958) *The Education of the Clinical Specialist in Psychiatric Nursing*, pp. 7–8, 18–22, 40–59. Reprinted in *The Clinical Nurse Specialist, Interpretations*, by J.P. Riehl & J.W. McVay (1973). Appleton Century Crofts, New York.

Nursing Development Conference Group (1973) *Concept Formalization in Nursing; Process and Product*. Little Brown & Co, Boston.

Padilla, G.V. (1972) The bases of the clinical nurse specialist's influence. *Hospital Progress*, April, 29–31.

Padilla, G.V. & Padilla, G.J. (1979) Nursing roles to improve patient care. *Nursing Digest*, **6** (4).

Reilly, J.A. (1976) Power persuasion. In: *Quality Patient Care and the Role of the Clinical Nursing Specialist* (ed. R. Rotkovitch). John Wiley & Sons, New York.

Reiter, F. (1961) Improvement of nursing practice. Reprinted paper in *The Clinical Nurse Specialist: Interpretations* (eds J.P. Riehl & J.W. McVay), 1973. Appleton Century Crofts, New York.

Report of Surgeon General's Consultant Group on Nursing (1963) US Public Health Service, *Toward Quality in Nursing: Needs and Goals* (Publication No. 992), p. 43. US Government Printing Office, Washington DC.

Rogers, M.E. (1970) *The Theoretical Basis of Nursing*. Lavis, Philadelphia.

Sample, S. (1975) The clinical specialist in a line position – a shared becoming. In: *The Clinical Nurse Specialist* – symposium, April. Sigma Theta Tau, Michigan, 1976.

Siegal, E. (1976) A versatile approach to supervision. In: *Quality Patient Care and the Role of the Clinical Nursing Specialist* (ed. R. Rotkovitch). John Wiley & Sons, New York.

Silver, H.K. *et al.* (1967) A program to increase health care for children and the paediatric nurse practitioner program. *Paediatrics*, **37**, 756–60.

Simms, L.L. (1973) Impact of patient centred approaches on the emergency role of the clinical nurse specialist. In: *New Directions in Patient Centred Nursing* (eds F.G. Abdellah *et al.*). Macmillan, New York.

Surgeon General's Consultant Group (1963) Follow up report. *American Journal of Nursing*, **67** (1), January, 1967.

Vaughan, M. (1968) Defining role of the clinical specialist. *Hospital Topics*, **5** (68), 93–4.

White, R. (1977) Mature of matutinal. *Nursing Mirror*, **144** (16), 41.

Chapter 3

Historical and Current Developments in Specialist and Advanced Practice in North America

Ann Hamric

Introduction

The development of specialized and advanced nursing practice in the USA has followed differing paths in its continuing evolution. Various terms, such as expanded roles, extended roles, specialization and advancement have been used to describe this practice evolution. This chapter will summarize the historical development of specialized nursing practice as distinguished from advanced nursing practice, with an emphasis on the clinical nurse specialist (CNS) and nurse practitioner (NP) roles. The practices of these two advanced practice nurse (APN) roles will be described. Current developments and issues will then be addressed. There is variability in both definition and role enactment of advanced nursing practice in the USA. Given the relatively recent development of the concept, this is not surprising. This chapter represents an overview of many complex roles and issues; interested readers are encouraged to review the references for more detail and discussion.

Historical development of specialists in nursing

Since the beginning of the twentieth century, American nurses with extensive experience and expertise in a selected area of nursing have considered themselves to be specialized (Hamric, 1989). In the first half of the twentieth century, hospitals offered 'postgraduate' courses in a variety of specialties. These courses included some specialty areas, such as dietetics, which actually left nursing to form new professions (Bullough, 1992). Because hospital-based diploma education was the standard preparation for professional nursing, these postgraduate courses were not formal education in the current understanding of the term. Instead, they generally involved informal, institutionally based classes with a strong apprenticeship approach (Bigbee, 1996).

Two of the earliest nursing specialties were nurse anesthesia and nurse-midwifery[1], both of which evolved from this type of training model. In the case of nurse anesthesia, advances in anesthetic agents and administration were important factors in the development of the role. In addition, physicians in the mid 1800s were interested in surgical procedures rather than anesthesia care. Nurses, often religious sisters who did not expect any payment, were recruited and trained to provide anesthesia care (Bigbee, 1996). Modern nurse-midwifery developed in response to identified needs for improved prenatal care in two areas of the USA, New York City and rural Kentucky. One of the major pioneers of the nurse-midwifery specialty was Mary Breckinridge, a registered nurse and British-trained midwife. She established the Frontier Nursing Service in Kentucky in 1925, which served as a model for later advanced practice development in primary care (Bigbee, 1996). The histories of these two specialties have been detailed by Thatcher (1953) for nurse anesthesia and Varney (1987) for nurse-midwifery, and will not be discussed here. It is important to note, however, that both specialties primarily developed outside mainstream American nursing.

Specialization involves concentration in a selected clinical area of nursing. The reality of modern nursing practice, and indeed of modern health care in general, is that all nurses are specialists to some extent. Even in public health settings, it is difficult to find a true generalist nurse; the knowledge base is too vast and clinical areas are themselves specialized. The term specialist also denotes a nurse who exhibits technical expertise. Peplau (1965) noted three social forces that preceded the development of areas of specialization:

(1)   Increasing information related to a specialty
(2)   Development of new technologies related to the specialty
(3)   Response to public interests and public need for the specialty.

One can see these three forces operating in the two specialties briefly noted above.

---

[1] Nurse anesthesia practice is distinguished by advanced procedural and pharmacological management of patients undergoing anesthesia. These APNs are known in the USA by the designation certified registered nurse anesthetist, or CRNA. Nurse-midwives use advanced health assessment and intervention skills to manage women's health and childbearing. They are known as certified nurse-midwives, or CNMs. Both specialties developed certification for practice at the advanced specialty level.

Nurses in the USA with extensive experience and continuing education in a particular clinical area of practice are eligible to become certified. Specialty certification examinations have been developed by specialty organizations such as the Emergency Nurses Association, the American Association of Critical Care Nurses and the Oncology Nursing Society, to recognize the development of specialty knowledge and skills. These examinations do not require completion of formal education beyond attaining the Registered Nurse license. The term 'nurse clinician' is commonly used to designate these nurses who have developed expert nursing skills based on extensive clinical experiences and informal study. Calkin (1984) designated these individuals as 'experts by experience' and contrasted them to advanced nursing practitioners.

Clinical nurse specialist (CNS)

Development of the CNS role

The preparation of a specialist in clinical nursing at the master's educational level represented a significant change from this traditional understanding of specialization (Hamric, 1989). While there is some disagreement about the origin of the CNS concept, the role was clearly developed to improve the quality of nursing care delivery by bringing a nurse with specialized experience and advanced formal education to the direct care interface. Peplau (1965) dated the title from 1938; in 1954 she developed the first master's program focused exclusively on psychiatric nursing practice. Reiter (1966) was also an early advocate of using graduate education programs to prepare nurses with advanced knowledge and clinical competence. Graduate educators became interested in the concept in the 1940s (Hamric, 1989). A strong surge of nurses returning from service during World War II were eligible for advanced education under the GI Bill (this bill was a federal government initiative to pay for the education of soldiers returning from the war). Also at this time, the US government appropriated funds for research and training for core mental health disciplines, which included psychiatric nursing. This specialty became the first to develop graduate level[2] clinical programs, with Peplau's program at Rutgers University in New Jersey.

A major impediment to the development of CNS programs was the

---

[2] In the USA, terminology for graduate education differs from that in the UK. Nurses with a bachelor's degree are referred to as having an undergraduate degree; in the UK, the term is graduate preparation. USA nurses with a master's degree are considered to have graduate level preparation; in the UK, the term post-graduate is used. Nurses with a doctoral degree are described similarly in both countries, although some discussions of graduate preparation in USA literature may include doctoral-level education as well as master's-level education.

prevailing assumption that education for nursing practice ended at the diploma level. Specialization in graduate education in the mid twentieth century consisted of programs for educators, supervisors, or administrators (Smoyak, 1976). As noted above, formal education for clinical practice was nonexistent. In 1963, the United States government expanded an important support program, the Professional Nurse Traineeship Program, to include CNS educational programs. This expansion of monetary support, the increasing number of baccalaureate-prepared nurses, and mainstream nursing's interest in formal graduate education, together firmly established CNS education at the graduate level. Burns *et al.* (1993) noted that 43.4% of the 175 master's level nursing programs they reviewed specifically prepared CNSs (an additional 11.4% prepared 'advanced clinicians'). Interestingly, a higher percentage of programs continued to prepare administrators (71.4%) and educators (62.8%).

Nursing leaders in the 1950s and 1960s believed that graduate education was the most efficient means of preparing CNSs. They also believed that developing nursing clinical education at the graduate level would increase nursing's professional status. These early advocates for the CNS concept were primarily a faculty in graduate nursing programs. Thus it is important to note that 'the CNS role was an innovation born out of mainstream nursing and enjoyed the strong support of nursing leaders' (Bigbee, 1996, p. 16). The CNS was conceived as an expert direct care provider who modeled advanced or newly developing practices to the general staff nurse. Thus, this role from its inception was firmly grounded in clinical practice. From the earliest days, however, the CNS concept included more than direct patient care. The role has always included education, consultation and research components in addition to expert practice (Georgopoulos & Christman, 1970). This broad conceptualization has been both a bane and a blessing. In their enthusiasm over the potential of the role, early writers broadly and enthusiastically described the CNS. This tendency to make the CNS 'all things to all people' has resulted in confusion about the CNS role, and widely differing practices (Hamric, 1989).

Description of CNS practice

From this brief history, it can be seen that even though both master's-prepared CNSs and nurses with extensive experience may consider themselves specialists, there are significant differences between the two groups of nurses. CNSs are nurses with a graduate degree (either master's or doctorate) who use expert knowledge and skills to improve the quality of patient care for a specialized patient population. They do this through direct expert practice to complex patients, through teaching and guiding clinical nursing staff to improve their care, through consulting within nursing and with other disciplines to improve care practices, and through utilizing and promoting research-based patient care practices (Hamric, 1989). The requirements of graduate education and the four sub-roles of practice, education, consultation and research are all important elements that distinguish the CNS from other specialized nurses. Some authors include administrative activities as a fifth sub-role (Tarsitano *et al.*, 1986; Hill *et al.*, 1993).

The National Association of Clinical Nurse Specialists (NACNS) has drafted a position statement on the CNS role (Lyon *et al.*, 1996) that describes the CNS as influencing patient care and care practices in three spheres: the patient/client/family sphere, the nursing and assistive staff sphere, and the organization/network sphere. This document emphasizes the CNS's mastery in actualizing nursing's unique and autonomous scope of practice through the 'diagnosis and treatment of non-disease-based causes of illness' (p. 3). Nursing oriented definitions of illness (as opposed to medical definitions) recognize that illness is a subjective experience that can be caused by factors other than disease. These factors include nausea, pain and functional or self-care problems such as skin breakdown, impaired mobility or confusion. These non-disease-based causes of illness clinically complicate a patient's course, and are frequently what make patients complex from a nursing standpoint. These are the areas in which CNSs are prepared to intervene. The NACNS statement also discusses the CNS's competencies in developing nursing practice and functioning as a clinical leader.

As one can see, the CNS role is multi-faceted and complex. The practice of a CNS is fluid and changes in response to changing patient and institutional needs. CNSs will not, and indeed probably should not, do the same thing year after year. In addition, no one CNS enacts all of the sub-roles simultaneously or possesses the skills and competencies equally. There is a strong developmental aspect to the role, and strong organizational skills and time management skills are necessary for success (Hamric, 1994). These factors make role definition an ongoing challenge for individual CNSs as well as the profession.

There has been much discussion in the USA's nursing literature about role ambiguity. The central definition of the CNS described above has not been consistently applied in all CNS practices, which has added to the confusion. The focus of the CNS's practice is on the patient/client and family, and this is an important distinguishing characteristic of all advanced practice nurses (Hamric, 1996; American Nurses Association (ANA), 1986). Regardless of setting or specialty, CNS practice is directed toward improving patient care and nursing practice for a group of patients and their families. One of the major problems that has occurred with the CNS role in some settings is its shifting away from a patient-focused practice. As one author noted:

'The use of clinical nurse specialists has often been predominantly for roles other than in-depth practice activities. In many ways, the specialist has been taken away from advanced expert practice and placed into roles related to special programming, delegated functional management, quality improvement activities, and education and development as well as a host of special projects and support activities. The problem with this is that the nurse in advanced clinical specialty practice should have a primary focus on patient care... The use of these practitioners for other activities has made it challenging to define specifically their value within the context of patient care.' (Porter-O'Grady, 1996, pp. 459–60)

One can see that using CNSs in the diverse ways described above has also greatly contributed to role confusion and misunderstanding about the CNS.

There is evidence of a growing consensus on the CNS role, however. Certainly this author's writings have attempted to be consistent in describing the CNS. Recent research demonstrated that staff nurses can have a clear and consistent understanding of the CNS role (Nuccio *et al.*, 1993). In this study, staff nurses in three hospitals in one city were surveyed concerning their perceptions of the CNS. There was little variability in the responses, with participants supporting the four sub-roles of practice, education, consultation and research as central elements of the CNS role. The NACNS position statement (Lyon *et al.*, 1996), currently in draft form being reviewed by the group's membership, represents an important consensus on the CNS role. Currently, CNSs comprise the largest APN group (Bigbee, 1996).

Nurse practitioner (NP)

Evolution of the NP role

In the 1960s and 1970s, an expanded or extended role of the NP developed in response to different dynamics from those creating the CNS role. Innovative practices in rural and occupational settings grew out of the roles of the public health nurse and nurse-midwife. Early attempts at role expansion did reflect a physician extender perspective. The physician assistant role[3] was introduced in the 1960s. Nursing leaders were critical of this role and contended that nurses were the more logical pro-

---

[3] Generally, physician assistants (PAs) are educated in undergraduate programs affiliated with schools of medicine. PAs are educated within a medical model to assist physicians and legally work under the supervision of a physician (Ballweg *et al.*, 1994). NPs, by contrast, work collaboratively with physicians and have independent legal accountability. NPs also provide advanced nursing care using a nursing model. NP programs require candidates to be registered nurses with baccalaureate degrees in nursing, while PA programs have broader entry criteria.

viders to assume expanded role activities in primary health care. Increasing emphasis on primary health care and social forces in the USA following the Vietnam War also fueled development of the NP role (Bigbee, 1996).

The early terminology referring to the NP as having an expanded or extended scope of practice indicated that the NP role encompassed practices from other disciplines, particularly medicine (Bigbee, 1996). Indeed, an acute shortage of primary care physicians in the 1960s and 1970s was a major impetus for NP development. The first NP program was developed in 1965 as a four-month certificate program jointly developed by a physician and a nurse to prepare pediatric NPs (Ford & Silver, 1967). As opposed to the CNS role, most early NP programs began outside schools of nursing because many nurse educators of that era questioned whether the NP was a valid nursing role. This lack of acceptance by educators was a barrier in developing mainstream graduate nursing education for the NP role (Bullough, 1992).

Early advocates were clear that they believed that the NP role would expand nursing's scope of practice to manage the *health* care of selected populations, not to change the nature of nursing or simply extend medical services (Ford, 1979). Early curricula were variable, owing to rapid program development and little consistency in academic standards (Bigbee, 1996). In some cases, NPs have been prepared to function as physician extenders rather than advanced nursing practitioners. In the past 20 years, there has been a notable shift to master's level preparation for nurse practitioners, although certificate programs continue to exist, particularly in the women's health area. In the early years, NPs were taught primarily by physicians rather than nursing faculty, but currently the NP program faculty consists generally of nurses who have developed NP skills. Certainly NP programs are now an accepted part of mainstream academic nursing education; in fact, these programs are proliferating rapidly in response to increasing demand for NPs. Programs have increased from 210 tracks offered in 73 institutions in 1992 to 372 tracks in 158 institutions by 1994 (Harper & Johnson, 1995).

Description of the NP role

The NP is a registered nurse who uses advanced assessment and diagnostic skills to care for patients. Most often, NPs deliver this care in primary health care settings in collaboration with physicians; this is the setting in which the role was conceived. NPs conduct physical examinations, diagnose and treat acute or chronic illnesses as well as minor injuries, and order and interpret lab tests and X-rays. In 47 of the USA's 50 states, they have some sort of prescriptive authority, although this varies between the states. As noted, while early educational programs for NPs were primarily certificate programs outside of schools of nursing, master's degree programs within nursing are now the norm for all NP programs.

NPs function primarily in direct patient care. Specialty areas with NP practice have developed, including pediatric, family, geriatric, women's health and acute care. Currently, there is particular interest in the acute care NP (Lott *et al*, 1996; Keane & Richmond, 1993). Nurse practitioners emphasize health and wellness, and do a great deal of anticipatory health counseling; they use a holistic approach and treat patients as partners in managing health care problems.

Traditionally, distinctions between NPs and CNSs were many, and some of these operate today. First, NPs generally functioned in primary care settings such as outpatient clinics or physician offices while CNSs functioned primarily in hospitals and tertiary medical centers. Second, CNSs were exclusively master's prepared in schools of nursing while NPs had a variety of educational tracks. Third, NPs had a broad range of physical, psychosocial and environmental assessment skills which they used to respond to common health and illness problems of the population for which they provide care. In contrast, CNSs had more selected competencies by virtue of their specialty focus. While CNSs may have had a narrower range of advanced assessment skills, they also had more depth in their ability to intervene with complex patient problems within their specialty population. Fourth, NPs usually focused entirely on direct patient care, while CNSs had additional sub-roles as part of their practice. Fifth, because NPs had medico-technical functions traditionally found in medical practice, some claimed they required more physician dependence and interdependence in both education and practice. CNSs, in contrast, were thought to be prepared and to practise exclusively in the tradition of nursing and thus were more independent of physician practice.

In the reality of today's current practice environment, many of these traditional distinctions are disappearing. These changes have been well discussed by Kitzman (1983, 1989), who argued that NPs are now primarily educated at the master's level within schools of nursing, as are CNSs. Both groups function collaboratively with physicians. Kitzman also demonstrated that CNSs are moving into primary care settings even as NPs are practising in acute care settings. Both groups generally learn a wide range of assessment skills and share many courses in graduate curricula. Indeed, the increasing similarities in educational preparation, in addition to the fact that NPs are providing care in hospitals and CNSs are providing care in primary care settings, have been major factors in the development of the core concept of advanced nursing practice to describe both of these practices. The similarities have also led some nursing leaders to advocate merging these two roles into one (Kitzman, 1989; Snyder & Mirr, 1995). Certainly, the blended CNS/NP role is a reality in some settings (Shuren, 1996).

Advanced nursing practice

The developing concept of advanced nursing practice

Bigbee (1996) noted that the evolution of the term 'advanced' in connection with nursing practice is unclear:

> 'Early in the evolution of the nurse practitioner role during the 1960s and 1970s, the term 'expanded' or 'extended' role was used throughout the literature, implying a horizontal movement to encompass expertise from medicine and other disciplines. The more contemporary term, 'advanced', suggests a more hierarchical movement encompassing increasing expertise within nursing rather than expansion into other disciplines.' (p. 4)

Although specialty practice is sometimes equated with advanced practice, increasingly the terms are distinguished from one another as described in this chapter. The term 'advanced practice nurse' is now widely used to delineate certified registered nurse anesthetists (CRNAs), certified nurse midwives (CNMs), CNSs and NPs. This trend has been given impetus by the American Nurses Association's[4] designation of these four roles as advanced practice (ANA, 1993), and by regulatory language in an increasing number of state nurse practice acts.

The concept of advanced nursing practice is still evolving in the USA, and various definitions exist in the nursing literature. It has been defined as any practice beyond the staff nurse role, a definition which would include nurse clinicians as well as APNs. Some authors define advanced nursing practice similarly to the ANA as practice in one of the four roles of CNS, NP, CNM and CRNA. One problem with this definition is that there are other APN roles in addition to these four; as advanced practice continues to evolve, it seems preferable to define advanced practice in other terms.

Over time, as the informal apprenticeship model of education for specialty practice has given way to formal educational programs housed within colleges and universities, consensus has emerged that preparation for advanced nursing practice should be at the master's level of education, and that this is an important distinguishing characteristic of the practice (AACN, 1995; ANA, 1995; Cronenwett, 1995; Hamric *et al.*, 1996; O'Malley *et al.*, 1996). A recent consensus statement from women's health NP leaders supporting matriculation to the master's degree is encouraging evidence that educational standardization for advanced practice is on the horizon (Hamric *et al.*, 1996).

In its latest social policy statement (ANA, 1995), the ANA defined

---

[4] The American Nurses Association is the national professional association for registered nurses in the USA.

advanced nursing practice as comprising three components: specialization, expansion and advancement:

> 'Specialization is concentrating or delimiting one's focus to part of the whole field of nursing. Expansion refers to the acquisition of new practice knowledge and skills, including the knowledge and skills that legitimize role autonomy within areas of practice that overlap traditional boundaries of medical practice. Advancement involves both specialization and expansion and is characterized by the integration of a broad range of theoretical, research-based, and practical knowledge that occurs as a part of graduate education in nursing.' (p. 14)

Hamric (1996) defined advanced nursing practice conceptually as 'the application of an expanded range of practical, theoretical and research-based therapeutics to phenomena experienced by patients within a specialized clinical area of the larger discipline of nursing' (p. 47). The term 'therapeutics' refers to any part of the nursing process, and recognizes that not all nursing therapeutics are research-based at this point in the profession's evolution. The critical importance of experiential and theoretical learning is emphasized, along with the patient-focused and specialized nature of the practice. Hamric further proposed defining characteristics of advanced nursing practice, comprised of primary criteria and core competencies (Fig. 3.1).

The primary criteria of graduate education, certification at an advanced level, and patient/family-focused practice are baseline criteria which constitute the core elements of advanced nursing practice. However, they are not sufficient to define the practice. The eight core competencies seen in Fig. 3.1 further define advanced nursing practice. These competencies mark advanced practice regardless of role function or setting. All of these defining elements function synergistically with characteristics of the individual APN to produce a unified composite practice that conforms to the conceptual definition – this is the essence of advanced nursing practice (Hamric, 1989).

Current status of advanced nursing practice

Both the understanding and the enactment of advanced nursing practice continue to evolve in the USA. Evolving roles such as the acute care NP (Lott *et al.*, 1996), the APN case manager (Mahn & Spross, 1996), and the blended CNS/NP role (Shuren, 1996) are increasingly visible and widely discussed. Societal pressures such as containment of health care costs, the shift to community-based managed care, changing legislative and regulatory climates in the different states, and continued escalating medical technology are creating unprecedented change and activity in health care settings (Hamric *et al.*, 1996). These factors result in considerable diversity in advanced practice opportunities in different settings and states. Differing

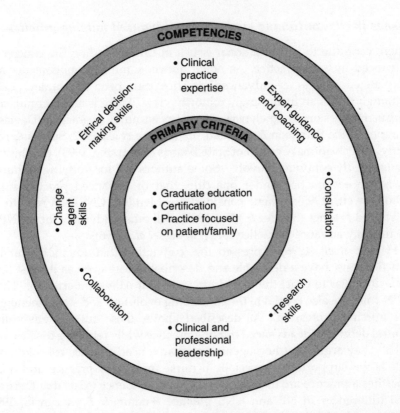

Fig. 3.1 Defining characteristics of advanced nursing practice (Reproduced with permission: Hamric, A.B. (1996) A definition of advanced nursing practice. In: *Advanced Nursing Practice: an integrative approach* (eds. A.B. Hamric, J.A. Spross and C.M. Hanson), p. 48. W.B. Saunders, Philadelphia.)

trends are occurring simultaneously. For example, CNS positions are being lost in some institutions in response to cost containment pressures. In other institutions, active hiring of CNSs is occurring. It is difficult to make any generalizations about the current state of advanced practice that would hold true throughout the USA. With this caveat, the following trends can be seen.

There is increased interest in and utilization of NPs, mainly in primary care settings but increasingly in acute care settings as well. As noted earlier, NP educational programs are experiencing the most rapid growth, but other APN programs are growing as well. There is concern that some schools are closing CNS programs in favor of preparing NPs exclusively (Lyon *et al.*, 1996). While noting that the future role of the CNS is receiving 'mixed reviews', Beecroft (1997) noted that emphasis on continuity of care, home care and job growth in non-hospital settings presents great possibilities for CNSs. All APNs are in situations of needing to financially justify their positions in terms of patient outcomes and cost containment. The need for research in these areas is frequently mentioned in the literature.

Issues in the continuing evolution of advanced nursing practice

There continue to be definitional issues in understanding the concept of advanced nursing practice. As noted above, some authors consider any specialized role to be advanced practice (Stimpson & Hanley, 1991), although this is an increasingly minority view. There is an emerging consensus on the core competencies of advanced nursing practice (Davies & Hughes, 1995; Patterson & Haddad, 1992; Price *et al.*, 1992; Spross & Baggerly, 1989; National Council of State Boards of Nursing, 1993), but this will undoubtedly continue to evolve. Some authors call for unifying all nurses in advanced practice under one title, that of advanced practice nurse (Cronenwett, 1995); others consider the blended CNS/NP role to be advanced practice (Snyder & Mirr, 1995); still others advocate for the NP to be the only advanced practice role (Hickey *et al.*, 1996).

Hamric *et al.* (1996) expressed the 'conviction that advanced nursing practice must have a definable and describable core even as it must have differing roles to enact the varied practices that APNs undertake ... These APN roles are also crucial to the continuing evolution and strengthening of the nursing profession'. As described above, these authors advocate a central definition of advanced nursing practice while retaining discrete role titles. They argue that homogenizing all advanced practice roles into one title is not supportable, especially if nurse midwifery practice and nurse anesthesia practice are included. In addition, evidence exists that there are real differences in NP and CNS practice (Fenton & Brykczynski, 1993; Williams & Valdivieso, 1994). Hamric *et al.* (1996) support use of the common title of APN for regulatory purposes, but retention of specific titles reflecting specific practices in health care settings. As they noted:

> 'Specific titles reflecting specific practices decrease confusion and enhance role clarity, especially when the role incumbents can clearly explain their practice and differentiate it from other APN practices. The public and policymakers can understand this distinction, just as they understand the term *physician* to be the overall descriptor of a medical professional, and *neurologist* or *cardiac surgeon* the descriptor of a physician in a particular specialty (see also Safriet, 1992).' (p. 609)

A second issue is the continuing evolution of new roles in advanced nursing practice. Particular examples include the acute care nurse practitioner and the APN case manager. The reality of these evolving roles is one reason Hamric (1996) developed a definition of advanced nursing practice that does not depend on particular role titles. The challenge is to be clear about the core understanding of advanced practice and how a new role such as case manager fits within that understanding. Without this clarity, there is risk that role confusion about advanced practice will actually be increased as new APN roles develop. It is also critical that as roles change and actual

APN practices become blended and merged, job titles should also change to reflect the actual practice. This is most especially seen in the blended CNS/NP role (Shuren, 1996).

Shuren described the blended CNS/NP as combining the primary health care skills of the NP with the in-depth, specialty knowledge of the CNS to enable expanded responsibilities for the more complex health problems experienced by patients in todays' health care system. Blended CNS/NP practice is characterized by work with a specialty patient population across primary, secondary and tertiary care settings, as well as involvement with nursing staff. As Shuren noted, 'The debate on merging CNS and NP curricula and skills to prepare one type of APN has overshadowed discussion and conceptualization of an APN who is jointly prepared as both a CNS and an NP' (p. 380). Perhaps this explains why the blended role has been slow to develop and why a satisfactory role title has not yet been agreed on.

A third issue receiving much attention in the USA is standardizing regulatory requirements across the states. In the USA, health care professionals are regulated at state level. The variation in APN regulation between the 50 different states is a major confusion and limitation on the development of advanced nursing practice. Specific differences include language in state nurse practice acts, certification requirements, level of prescriptive authority allowed, and availability of reimbursement for practice (Hanson, 1996). Readers interested in more detail on this issue are referred to the writings of Hanson, Safriet (1992), and O'Malley *et al.* (1996).

A fourth issue for all health care professionals is the continuing changes in health care delivery in the USA. Particular marketplace reforms include development of managed care systems and the shift to out-patient care delivery. O'Malley *et al.* (1996) described the evolution of the USA system as moving from a specialty care, illness-focused, single institution model to a model emphasizing primary care, health and lifestyle management, and integrated networks of institutions and providers. They asserted that these changes 'have created an array of exciting opportunities for nurses engaged in advanced practice' (p. 63), even while noting that lack of understanding of APN roles has meant that the actual and potential contributions of APNs in these evolving care delivery models have not yet been fully realized.

Finally, a fifth issue of great importance within the nursing community in the USA is the need for nursing's internal cohesion. This is a tremendous challenge because there are many voices speaking to advanced nursing practice, and as has been seen, they do not all agree. There are in addition numerous specialty organizations with competing and sometimes opposing interests which further the disunity within the profession about the concept of advanced practice. Important coalition building is occurring in relation to NP education (Hamric *et al.*, 1996), and needs to extend to all APN groups. The ability to work collectively on articulating advanced practice, clarifying APN education and practice, and addressing policy and regulatory issues is essential to ensuring a viable future for all APN roles.

Conclusion

The history of advanced practice in nursing as distinguished from specialty practice is a recent development in the overall history of the nursing profession. As such, it is continuing to evolve amid ever-increasing changes in the health care system of the USA. 'These are years of great promise and great risk for APNs' (Hamric *et al.*, 1996). Even with this brief history, one can see that advanced nursing practitioners have been characterized by their flexibility and creativity in responding to needs of the health-care system. These characteristics, along with greater clarity and consistency in preparation and role enactment, can lead to continued evolution and diversification of advanced nursing practice.

References

AACN (1995) *The essentials of master's education for advanced practice nursing.* Report from the task force on the essentials of master's education for advanced practice nursing. American Association of Colleges of Nursing, Washington DC.

ANA (1986) *The Role of the Clinical Nurse Specialist.* American Nurses Association, Council of Clinical Nurse Specialists, Kansas City.

ANA (1993) *Advanced Practice Nursing: A New Age in Health Care, Nursing Facts.* American Nurses Publishing, American Nurses Association, Washington DC.

ANA (1995) *Nursing's Social Policy Statement.* American Nurses Association, Washington DC.

Ballweg, R., Stolberg, S. & Sullivan, E.M. (1994) *Physician Assistant: A Guide to Clinical Practice.* W.B. Saunders, Philadelphia.

Beecroft, P.C. (1997) CNSs' future role in healthcare. *Clinical Nurse Specialist*, **11**, 143.

Bigbee, J.L. (1996) History and evolution of advanced nursing practice. In: *Advanced Nursing Practice: an Integrative Approach* (eds A.B. Hamric, J.A. Spross & C.M. Hanson), pp. 3–24. W.B. Saunders, Philadelphia.

Bullough, B. (1992) Alternative models for specialty nursing practice. *Nursing and Health Care*, **13**, 254–9.

Burns, P., Nishikawa, H., Weatherby, F., Forni, P., Moran, M., Allen, M., Baker, C. & Brooten, D. (1993) Masters degree nursing education: state of the art. *Journal of Professional Nursing*, **9**, 267–76.

Calkin, J.D. (1984) A model for advanced nursing practice. *Journal of Nursing Administration*, **14** (1), 24–30.

Cronenwett, L. (1995) Molding the future of advanced practice nursing. *Nursing Outlook*, **43** (3), 112–18.

Davies, B. & Hughes, A.M. (1995) Clarification of advanced nursing practice: characteristics and competencies. *Clinical Nurse Specialist*, **9**, 156–60.

Fenton, M.V. & Brykczynski, K.A. (1993) Qualitative distinctions and similarities in the practice of clinical nurse specialists and nurse practitioners. *Journal of Professional Nursing*, **9**, 313–26.

Ford, L. (1979) A nurse for all settings: the nurse practitioner. *Nursing Outlook*, **27**, 516–21.

Ford, L. & Silver, H. (1967) Expanded role of the nurse in child care. *Nursing Outlook*, **15**, 43–5.

Georgopoulos, B.S. & Christman, L. (1970) The clinical nurse specialist: a role model. *American Journal of Nursing*, **70**, 1030–39.

Hamric, A.B. (1989) History and overview of the CNS role. In: *The Clinical Nurse Specialist in Theory and Practice* (eds A.B. Hamric & J.A. Spross), 2nd edn, pp. 3–18. W.B. Saunders, Philadelphia.

Hamric, A.B. (1994) History and overview of the clinical nurse specialist role. *Japanese Journal of Nursing Research*, **27** (5), 33–45.

Hamric, A.B. (1996) A definition of advanced nursing practice. In: *Advanced Nursing Practice: An Integrative Approach* (eds A.B. Hamric, J.A. Spross & C.M. Hanson), pp. 42–56. W.B. Saunders, Philadelphia.

Hamric, A.B., Spross, J.A. & Hanson, C.M. (1996) Surviving system and professional turbulence. In: *Advanced Nursing Practice: an integrative approach* (eds A.B. Hamric, J.A. Spross & C.M. Hanson), 2nd edn, pp. 601–19. W.B. Saunders, Philadelphia.

Hanson, C.M. (1996) Health policy issues: dealing with the realities and constraints of advanced nursing practice. In: *Advanced Nursing Practice: An Integrative Approach* (eds A.B. Hamric, J.A. Spross & C.M. Hanson), pp. 496–516. W.B. Saunders, Philadelphia.

Harper, D. & Johnson, J. (1995) *Interim preliminary report of the workforce policy project: comparison of the 1992 to 1994 national nurse practitioner program directories*. Paper presented at the annual conference of the National Organization of Nurse Practitioner Faculties National Conference, Denver.

Hickey, J.V., Ouimette, R.M. & Venegoni, S.L. (1996) *Advanced Practice Nursing: Changing Roles and Clinical Applications*. Lippincott, Philadelphia.

Hill, K.M., Ellsworth-Wolk, J. & DeBlase, R. (1993) Capturing the multiple contributions of the CNS role: a criterion-based evaluation tool. *Clinical Nurse Specialist*, **4**, 267–73.

Keane, A. & Richmond, T. (1993) Tertiary NPs. *Image: The Journal of Nursing Scholarship*, **25** (4), 281–4.

Kitzman, H.J. (1983) The CNS and the nurse practitioner. In: *The Clinical Nurse Specialist in Theory and Practice* (eds A.B. Hamric & J.A. Spross), pp. 275–90. Grune & Stratton, New York.

Kitzman, H.J. (1989) The CNS and the nurse practitioner. In: *The Clinical Nurse Specialist in Theory and Practice* (eds A.B. Hamric and J.A. Spross), 2nd edn, pp. 379–94. W.B. Saunders, Philadelphia.

Lott, J.W., Polak, J.D., Kenyon, T.B. & Kenner, C.A. (1996) Acute care nurse practitioner. In: *Advanced Nursing Practice: An integrative approach* (eds A.B. Hamric, J.A. Spross & C.M. Hanson), pp. 351–74. W.B. Saunders, Philadelphia.

Lyon, B.L., Davidson, S., Beecroft, P.C., Bingle, J., Dayhoff, N. & Ellstrom, K. (1996)

Statement on clinical nurse specialist practice and education. Working document No. 2, National Association of Clinical Nurse Specialists, Aliso Viejo, California.

Mahn, V.A. & Spross, J.A. (1996) Nurse case management as an advanced practice role. In: *Advanced Nursing Practice: an Integrative Approach* (eds A.B. Hamric, J.A. Spross & C.M. Hanson), pp. 445–67. W.B. Saunders, Philadelphia.

National Council of State Boards of Nursing (1993) *Position paper on the regulation of advanced nursing practice.* National Council of State Boards of Nursing, Chicago.

Nuccio, S.A., Costa-Lieberthal, K.M., Gunta, K.E. *et al.* (1993) A survey of 636 staff nurses: perceptions and factors influencing the CNS role. *Clinical Nurse Specialist,* **7,** 122–8.

O'Malley, J., Cummings, S. & King, C.S. (1996) The politics of advanced practice. *Nursing Administration Quarterly,* **20** (3), 62–72.

Patterson, C. & Haddad, B. (1992) The advanced nurse practitioner: common attributes. *Canadian Journal of Nursing Administration,* **5** (3), 18–22.

Peplau, H.E. (1965) Specialization in professional nursing. *Nursing Science,* **3,** 268–87.

Porter-O'Grady, T. (1996) A glimpse over the horizon: the future of advanced practice nursing. In: *Nursing Management in the New Paradigm* (eds C.E. Loveridge & S.H. Cummings), pp. 456–94. Aspen, Gaithersburg.

Price, M.J., Martin, A.C., Newberry, Y.G., Zimmer, P.A., Brykczynski, K.A. & Warren, R. (1992) Developing national guidelines for nurse practitioner education: an overview of the product and the process. *Journal of Nursing Education,* **31** (1), 10–15.

Reiter, F. (1966) The nurse-clinician. *American Journal of Nursing,* **66,** 274–80.

Safriet, B.J. (1992) Health care dollars and regulatory sense: the role of advanced practice nursing. *Yale Journal of Regulation,* **9,** 417–87.

Shuren, A.W. (1996) The blended role of the clinical nurse specialist and the nurse practitioner. In: *Advanced Nursing Practice: An Integrative Approach* (eds A.B. Hamric, J.A. Spross & C.M. Hanson), pp. 375–94. W.B. Saunders, Philadelphia.

Smoyak, S.A. (1976) Specialisation in nursing: from then to now. *Nursing Outlook,* **24,** 676–81.

Snyder, M. & Mirr, M.P. (1995) *Advanced Practice Nursing: A Guide to Professional Development.* Springer Publishing, New York.

Spross, J.A. & Baggerly, J. (1989) Models of advanced practice. In: *The Clinical Nurse Specialist in Theory and Practice* (eds A.B. Hamric & J.A. Spross), 2nd edn, pp. 19–40. W.B. Saunders, Philadelphia.

Stimpson, M. & Hanley, B. (1991) Nurse policy analyst: advanced practice role. *Nursing and Health Care,* **12** 10–15.

Tarsitano, B.J., Brophy, E.B. & Snyder, D.J. (1986) A demystification of the clinical nurse specialist role: perceptions of clinical nurse specialists and nurse administrators. *Journal of Nursing Education,* **25** (1), 4–9.

Thatcher, V.S. (1953) *A History of Anesthesia: With Emphasis on the Nurse Specialist.* J.B. Lippincott, Philadelphia.

Varney, H. (1987) *Nurse-midwifery,* 2nd edn. Blackwell Science, Boston.

Williams, C.A. & Valdivieso, G.C. (1994) Advanced practice models: a comparison of clinical nurse specialist and nurse practitioner activities. *Clinical Nurse Specialist,* **8,** 311–18.

Chapter 4

Legal Issues for Advanced and Specialist Nurse Practitioners

John Tingle

Introduction

Nurses today are practising in an environment where patients are increasingly resorting to litigation and to making formal complaints. The NHS cannot ignore such facts, and risk management strategies dealing with avoiding complaints and litigation have been introduced by many health authorities and trusts. These strategies deal with such matters as improving communication with patients, analysing complaints and adverse incidents, clinical risk management, benchmarking, complaint handling, clinical pathways and guidelines, education programmes introducing clinical negligence actions and many other issues.

Nurses who are redefining their practice are having to work in a care environment which is having to respond to these strategies and the general care environment as described above. This chapter discusses this new environment of care and looks at a number of key legal and professional accountability issues. Best practice, problems in communicating with patients and others and record keeping will be discussed. The concept of legal competence will be discussed particularly within the context of nurses performing expanded roles and evidence based practice. Advice from the professional bodies on these matters will be discussed.

It will be seen that communication failures lie at the heart of many complaints and court cases. The adoption of good communication strategies is an essential prerequisite of good professional reflective practice and of the exercise of patient advocacy.

Complaints and litigation

It seems that the general public are now much better informed about health care rights generally and have a greater sense of entitlement. Initiatives such as *The Patients Charter* and the publicity given to reported cases have raised expectations and knowledge levels. The Health Service Commissioner (HSC, 1997–8) or ombudsman has reported another record year of complaints. In the period 1996–7 the HSC received 2219 complaints, 24% up on the previous year; 93% of complaints about complaint handling by health authorities or Trusts were upheld by the HSC. The overall upheld grievance figure was 63%. Matters complained of included failures in communication, consent and counselling, privacy, breach of confidence, complaint handling and so on.

While some patients' complaints are dealt with under hospital complaints procedures and the HSC, others may proceed to formal court hearings if the patient feels that they have been the subject of negligent treatment and they have suffered injury as a result.

The litigation levels for clinical negligence are increasing significantly each year. The NHS Executive (1996a) state:

> 'The total cost of NHS clinical negligence is currently estimated at around £200 million, and is likely to grow at nearly 25% per annum over the next 5 years, of which the share directly borne by Trusts will rise from about 10% to 75%.'

According to the NHS Executive (1996b) the projected total cost of clinical negligence in the year 2000–1 will be around £500 million. They explain that:

> 'Although such projections are inevitably somewhat uncertain, the general pattern of increasing costs is likely to be a reflection of:
> (i)   increases in the volume of NHS activity;
> (ii)   the increasing tendency for patients to seek redress when incidents occur; and
> (iii) continuing upward pressures on the size of negligence awards over and above the general level of litigation.'

Health authority, Trust and HSC investigations and court proceedings can directly involve specialist and advanced nurse practitioners as witnesses or as potential defendants.

Why do patients sue and complain?

There has been some research in this area which supports the direct practical experiences of many health lawyers and clinicians that often patients simply required an explanation of what occurred to them, an apology and an assurance that it would not happen to anybody else. Patients have not received this information and have resorted to making formal complaints and sometimes approaching solicitors.

Action for Victims of Medical Accidents (AVMA, 1995) states:

'The vast majority of patients who have experienced something going wrong during medical care, or their relatives if the patient has died, are not interested in compensation. Money cannot compensate, for example, for the loss of a child or another loved one or for the loss of health. What they want is "satisfaction". What that means is a full explanation of what went wrong, an honest explanation of why it went wrong and, if appropriate, an apology for what actually happened. They will also want to be assured that all steps will be taken to ensure that a similar accident does not happen to someone else in the future. Of course, there are times when financial compensation is also necessary and that will form part of the "satisfaction" that the patient wants.'

Vincent *et al.*'s (1994) study supports the AVMA conclusions. The authors examined the reasons patients and their relatives take legal action and surveyed 227 patients and their relatives who were taking legal action through five firms of plaintiff medical negligence solicitors. They found that the decision to take legal action was determined not only by the original injury, but also by insensitive handling and poor communication after the original incident:

'Four main factors were identified in the analysis of reasons for litigation...
- accountability – wish to see staff disciplined and called to account;
- explanation – a combination of wanting an explanation and feeling ignored or neglected after the incident;
- standards of care – wishing to ensure that a similar incident did not happen again; and
- compensation – wanting compensation and an admission of negligence.'

Where explanations were given for the incidents, fewer than 15% were considered satisfactory.

The Wilson Committee report on the NHS complaints procedures (DoH, 1994) discussed the objectives of complainants and noted that it was rare for a complainant to be motivated by prejudice or malice. Some complainants may show signs of severe mental disorder and some complaints can be made out of feelings of grief or guilt. There is a high proportion of complaints following bereavement. Complainants want to be taken seriously.

It is necessary to determine the underlying causes of these problems in order to try and effect some positive changes. The Audit Commission (1993) conclude on the underlying causes of poor clinical communication:

'Patients and relatives often do not get enough information, the communication process is poorly handled and it is conducted in unsympathetic environments. Instead of their needs driving the process, it is shaped by underlying problems in the management and organisation of clinical services... These include:
- poor communication between clinical staff;

- an approach to communication based mainly on clinicians' subjective views; and
- a gap between clinical work and general management.'

These studies show that specialist and advanced practitioner nurses must be aware of the need to maintain good communication practices with patients and to ensure that strategies are in place to manage properly untoward incidents. It is also important to remember that saying sorry does not mean you are admitting legal liability.

These studies provide us with an awareness of the communication problems that exist. The issues are out in the open to be discussed and acted upon by nurses and others. How well these issues are dealt with will be revealed over the course of time as new studies are commissioned and HSC reports hopefully begin to identify significant improvements taking place. Some strategies for improving communication are discussed below.

As well as good patient communication skills good records are also essential in order to provide safe reflective practice.

Record keeping

Complaints and court cases may proceed a good number of months or even years (with court cases) after the treatment. Memories fade with the passage of time and the written record often remains the only reliable, tangible record of events. Records also form an essential part of the care process. The nursing process itself is dependent on recording. Clinical, audit and clinical risk management strategies also run on records and their effectiveness is wholly dependent on their quality.

Furthermore, the specialist and advanced nurse practising expanded roles have to meet a high level of legal accountability. In carrying out expanded roles nurses may be expected to demonstrate the knowledge and skills that a doctor would have of the activity if it was normally performed by a doctor. This is seen in terms of the legal standard of care which the courts may expect, and will be discussed below. Protocols and other records are important in establishing that a safe and reflective environment of care was being practised.

Many argue that nurse record keeping could be greatly improved and stricter procedures for nursing records are being prepared by the UK government under the leadership of England's chief nurse, Yvonne Moore (*Nursing Standard*, 1997). The Audit Commission (1992) and the HSC have noted problems with nursing records:

'The Audit Commission's examination of patient records confirms the Ombudsman's view of record-keeping in nursing as "ritualistic", and lacking essential information...

Problems with nursing records:
- records undated and unsigned
- lack of detail about the person rather than the medical problem
- insufficient information about the patient's perception of the problem, and response to treatment
- patient's psychological and emotional needs not documented
- objectives for care not established
- progress towards care objectives not evaluated
- assessments for discharge and discharge plans not documented.

Nurses need greater incentives to invest the time and energy that care planning requires. Specifically, they need to be able to feel the benefits of doing it properly. They need to be able to develop professionally through writing comprehensive, detailed care plans, seeing the outcomes of their own clinical decisions, learning from their mistakes and judging the quality of their planning skills.'

Record keeping problems are not confined to the nursing profession. The medical profession has similar problems. The Audit Commission (1995) stated that a defensible record needs to be legible, accurate, timely and comprehensive and that more than a quarter of doctors' notes (history sheets) failed this test.

Record keeping problems have been clearly identified and they need to be fully addressed. In patient care, if some form of treatment or observation was not recorded, there exists a real danger it may be deemed never to have taken place. An old legal adage applies: poor records poor defence, no records no defence.

Having identified the problems it is necessary to advance some solutions.

Making improvements

Improving communications

Advice on improving patient communication comes from many quarters and can often be seen as applied common sense. It is valuable because it may emanate from outside organizations which can put fresh perspectives on issues. The Audit Commission (1993) have provided useful advice on improving communication. Advice has also been issued by the Royal College of Physicians of London (1997). The advice can be usefully applied to advanced and specialist nurses. Guidelines are given for a good communication strategy:

'(1) Provide the most important information first – good news before bad
(2) Explain how each item of information will affect the patient personally
(3) Present information in separate categories
(4) Make advice specific, detailed and concrete

(5) Use words the patient knows or define unfamiliar words. Write down key words and unfamiliar words, draw a diagram, and keep a copy

(6) Repeat the information, using the same words each time, and prepare material, written or taped, to back up the handwritten note.'

The UKCC (1996a) offer useful advice on communicating and state:

'To ensure that you gain the trust of your patients and clients, you should recognise them as equal partners, use language that is familiar to them and make sure that they understand the information that you are giving.'

Good communication skills also underpin the new hospital complaints procedure and are essential for its effective implementation (NHS Executive, 1996c).

Inextricably linked with patient communication skills and strategies are record keeping skills and strategies.

Improving records

A statutory scheme for managing complaints and litigation, the Clinical Negligence Scheme for Trusts (CNST, 1996; NHS Executive, 1996a) has risk management standards which include complaints and record keeping. The CNST is a voluntary scheme enabling Trusts to pool the costs of clinical negligence settlements each year in return for an annual contribution. There is a direct financial incentive for Trusts to satisfy the standards as they can obtain discounts on their annual contribution to the scheme (Pincombe, 1996).

The Audit Commission (1995) report contains a great deal of useful advice on good practice principles and the pitfalls of record keeping. Key recommendations include:

'Hospitals should agree a "case note architecture" setting out the optimal content and order of case notes.

They should provide clear guidelines and standards for all their staff, including doctors, based on professional good practice. Performance against these standards should be monitored.

They should aim, so far as possible, to have only one set of case notes for each patient.'

Green *et al.* (1996) of the Medical Defence Union (MDU) discuss medical records and provide a useful strategy:

'Accurate, complete and contemporaneous medical records can help to refute complaints and claims. They ensure continuity of care and treatment within the primary healthcare team. It is wise to make an entry in the medical record after every:

- consultation
- visit
- telephone conversation
- out-of-hours communication

Important negative findings should also be noted.'

UKCC (1993) advice on records and record keeping provides an important focus on these issues and topics considered include the purpose and importance of records, standards for records, the legal status of records and its implications, and so on.

Some sources of advice on communication and record keeping have been highlighted. The specialist and advanced nurse practitioner, as part of his or her professional and legal accountability, must be aware of the problems that generally exist with communications and record keeping in health care. To act effectively as the reflective practitioner and a patient advocate the nurse should maintain high standards in all these areas.

Nurses are professionals and as such are legally and professionally accountable to their patients for any actions or omissions which result in harm. In the next section there is a discussion on the legal and professional accountability of nurses with particular reference to the specialist and advanced practitioner.

Legal competence and clinical risk management

The competence of a specialist and advanced nurse may be tested in the courts if a patient alleges that the nurse was negligent and that because of this, harm resulted to the patient. Such a case is reported by the *Nursing Standard* (1996):

> 'Professor Martin said a nurse had already been held to be negligent in an unreported case because she had failed to pick up signs of infection that a doctor would have spotted.'

In the present litigious care environment it looks likely that more cases involving specialist and advanced practitioner nurses will arise. Goodwin and Moss (1997), in discussing clinical risk in A&E nursing, state:

> 'The introduction and development of the nurse practitioner role in A&E has combined some of the duties of the senior nurse and junior doctor. As a result, nurse practitioners are now more likely to be subject to complaints and allegations of negligence... The only way of looking at the possible types of claim that nurse practitioners may face is by reviewing previous cases with junior hospital doctors. Historically, this group has been implicated in a variety of medical negligence claims.'

The fear of litigation and complaints is a fact of everyday life for all professions. One possible solution is to adopt clinical risk management strategies that can help manage risks. Clinical risk management at its most basic is simply applied common sense: a strategy put into place to avoid an untoward event occurring. The term has no absolute meaning and is a very fluid concept. The communication and record keeping strategies discussed above are examples of the application of clinical risk management, as are staff legal and professional accountability awareness programmes and discussions. The concept underpins the CNST (NHS Executive, 1996a) and other centralized health quality litigation management programmes.

It is interesting to speculate whether the following adverse incidents given by Mark Jones RCN, community adviser, and quoted by Waters (1996), would have arisen if the health carers involved had been aware of the nature and extent of their professional and legal accountabilities, particularly legal expectations of their competence and of the practical need to manage risk through effective clinical risk management strategies.

> '... one case where a practice nurse with no formal midwifery training had taken over antenatal care and had missed a fetus dying in utero ... Poor communication at another surgery led to a practice nurse accidentally giving a rubella vaccination to a woman who was three months pregnant. She had come to the surgery worried about being exposed to the virus and the receptionists had squeezed her into the nurse "immunisation clinic" ...'

A court considering the cases above would need to determine the standard of legal care to be expected from the nurse in the situations given, which would be a question of law. The nurse would, on the judicial precedents that will be discussed below, be assumed to have the knowledge of the professionals who traditionally perform those activities. In the cases above, experts would be consulted by the lawyers and their advice would probably be that midwives and doctors would normally perform the clinical activities. Clearly it is difficult in practice to pinpoint the boundaries of medical and nursing practice as there is shift and overlap. What were once medical activities can over time be absorbed into nursing.

In the cases above and where nurses are doing activities that are generally dealt with by other professionals it will be seen that their skill and knowledge base will be expected by the court to correspond with that of those other professionals. Nurses performing endoscopies (Hughes, 1996) would be expected to demonstrate medical skills and knowledge.

Negligence

The tort of negligence is composed of a number of parts:

(1)   A legal duty to take reasonable care

(2)   Breach of that duty
(3)   Reasonably foreseeable damage caused to the plaintiff because of the breach.

Proof

All the above elements must be in place before a patient can sue. The burden of proving the case, on the civil standard of proof not the higher criminal standard, falls on the plaintiff. Sometimes, however, the negligence may be obvious, for example where forceps may be left in a patient. In these circumstances the burden of proof remains with the plaintiff but the defendant must adduce evidence to rebut the inference of negligence, in order to avoid a finding of liability (Jones, 1996). Lawyers use the maxim, '*Res ipsa loquitur*', meaning 'the thing speaks for itself'.

Duty

The issue of owing a duty of care is not generally a problematic issue in malpractice cases. The law focuses on such concepts as foreseeability of harm, proximity of relationship, voluntary assumption of responsibility and public policy in deciding whether a duty of legal care is owed. There is no doubt that nurses owe their patients a legal duty of care. The issue of breach of duty is likely to be more problematic (Jones, 1996).

Breach of duty

The standard of care to be exercised by the nurse, and whether he or she has fallen below that standard, will be a central issue in any malpractice case. The Bolam principle is the classic test of professional competence and is a prime source of medical and nursing legal accountability. The test comes from the case of *Bolam* v. *Friern Hospital Management Committee* [1957] 2 All ER 118. Mr Justice McNair stated the following important principles which apply to all professionals:

'The test is the standard of the ordinary skilled man exercising and professing to have that special skill. A man need not possess the highest expert skill at the risk of being found negligent. It is well established law that it is sufficient if he exercises the ordinary skill of an ordinary competent man exercising that particular art.

A doctor is not guilty of negligence if he has acted in accordance with a practice accepted as proper by a responsible body of medical men skilled in that particular art... Putting it the other way round, a doctor is not negligent, if he is acting in accordance with such a practice, merely because there is a body of opinion that takes a contrary view. At the same time, that does not mean that a medical man can obstinately and pig-headedly carry on with some old technique if it has been proved to be contrary to what is really substantially the whole of informed medical opinion.'

Nurses like all other professionals must act reasonably. The legal competence level is that of the ordinary skilled nurse, not the best or the worst. Nurses can disagree about treatments and, under Bolam, minority nursing views and opinions can be viewed as being proper. The judge, however, has the final say on these matters.

The concept of evidenced-based nursing and medicine practice may in time have some influence and affect the Bolam principle. If most health carers practise evidenced-based nursing or medicine, best practice may be more appropriate to look for as the proper standard.

Causation

Another key issue to determine is that the nurse's negligence made some difference to the plaintiff. If the negligence has not caused or materially contributed to the plaintiff's damage, there can be no claim.

The objective standard of care

The standard of care expected of the reasonable doctor or nurse is objective. The courts consider what the ordinary skilled nurse in the relevant speciality would have done in the circumstances of the case. When people are filling in other roles, learning tasks or doing activities traditionally done by others, the courts approach the issue of competence in the same objective way. Jones (1996) summarizes the approach:

'It is axiomatic that the standard of care expected of the reasonable man is objective, not subjective. It eliminates the personal equation and takes no account of the particular idiosyncrasies or weaknesses of the defendant. Thus, the defendant who is inexperienced or who is just learning a particular task must come up to the standard of the reasonably competent and experienced person. His "incompetent best" is not good enough. This principle applies with as much force to an inexperienced doctor as it does to an inexperienced motorist.'

Two recent cases illustrate the applicable principles which would apply equally to specialist and advanced nurses. The first is *Wilsher* v. *Essex Area Health Authority* [1986] 3 All ER 801.

The plaintiff was an infant child who was born prematurely suffering from various illnesses, including oxygen deficiency. While the plaintiff was in the unit a junior and inexperienced doctor monitoring the oxygen in the plaintiff's bloodstream mistakenly inserted a catheter into a vein rather than an artery, but then asked the senior registrar to check what he had done. Unfortunately he failed to see the mistake and made the same error some time later himself when replacing the catheter. As a result the plaintiff was given excess oxygen and sued alleging that this had caused an incurable condition of the retina which resulted in blindness. The case was eventually settled with the health authority paying compensation.

A number of key legal issues were discussed in the case, which included the content of the standard of care of the junior doctor. Lord Justice Mustill said:

> 'For my part, I prefer the third of the propositions which have been canvassed. This relates the duty of care, not to the individual, but to the post which he occupies. I would differentiate "post" from "rank" or "status". In a case such as the present, the standard is not just of the averagely competent and well-informed junior houseman (or whatever the position of the doctor) but of such a person who fills a post in a unit offering a highly specialised service.'

Lord Justice Glidewell stated:

> 'In my view, the law requires the trainee or learner to be judged by the same standard as his more experienced colleagues. If it did not, inexperience would frequently be urged as a defence to an action for professional negligence.'

The junior doctor in this case was not found to be negligent as he had done the reasonable thing by asking the registrar what to do. The registrar was found to be in breach of his duty of care.

The Wilsher case was followed in *Djemal* v. *Bexley Health Authority* [1995] 6 Med LR 269. This case involved a senior house officer in A&E who failed to make a proper diagnosis of a patient who presented with a severe sore throat. The doctor diagnosed that the plaintiff was suffering from a viral upper respiratory tract infection and prescribed gargling with aspirin and the use of a spray. He sent the patient home, but he returned later to hospital in a very bad condition. He suffered a respiratory arrest and a diagnosis was subsequently made that the plaintiff had suffered hypoxic brain damage. He remained in a persistent vegetative state. The hospital notes recorded that the plaintiff had a severe obstructive epiglottis.

The senior house officer was found to be negligent in failing to notice the plaintiff's spitting and pooling of saliva due to inability to swallow. He failed to obtain a proper history and consequently failed to obtain information which would have induced a reasonably competent casualty officer to have retained the patient for further investigation by others. The judge, Sir Haydn Tudor Evans, said:

> 'The test applied to the facts is that of a reasonably competent senior houseman acting as a casualty officer without any reference to the length of experience. The test to be applied is that adopted by the majority of the Court of Appeal in *Wilsher* v. *Essex Area Health Authority* ...'

From these judicial precedents we can derive a number of principles which have been discussed earlier. Specialist and advanced nurses may well be expected to demonstrate medical skills and knowledge. Their legal standard of care can be set at a medical level.

The courts have said that inexperience is no defence to clinical malpractice and look to the post occupied and the tasks performed to establish the standard of care to be expected. They would also look to see whether a reflective environment of care was in operation. Protocols which deal with the medical tasks being performed are evidence of this and are a fundamental aspect of the clinical risk management process. Guidelines from the UKCC (1992a,b, 1996) and other professional medical organisations (GMC, 1995; BMA, 1996) could also be considered in court.

Expanded role guidelines: divergent views

A court considering a case of nursing negligence against a specialist or advanced nurse will be understandably confused by the advice which has emanated from the professional organizations on the topic of expanded role. There is no consensus between medical (GMC, 1995; BMA, 1996) and nursing guidance (UKCC, 1992a; 1996) and this could result in communication and accountability problems. Dowling *et al.* (1996) state:

'When analysed together and compared, the regulations arising from the professional bodies (GMC and UKCC), civil law concerning certain wrongs to patients, and employment law are sometimes contradictory and hard to interpret. The resulting uncertainties about appropriate management for clinical roles evolving *between* the professions, coupled with an increasingly litigious public, put the nurses and consultants involved at risk of complaints and of disciplinary and legal action.'

The UKCC position

The main UKCC statement on expanded role is *The Scope of Professional Practice* (UKCC, 1992a). This document gives emphasis to and focuses on the individual accountability of the nurse for professional practice. The UKCC state that the principles set out in paragraphs 8 to 10 inclusive provide 'the basis for ensuring that practice remains dynamic and is able readily and appropriately to adjust to meet changing care needs'. These principles respect and recognize the individual and professional autonomy of the nurse to make decisions about the appropriate scope of his or her professional practice. (UKCC 1992b, 1996)

GMC and BMA guidance appears to view matters differently and maintain the basic premise of doctor delegation and responsibility for medical skills that nurses may carry out. Their guidance appears very prescriptive and doctor centred. The GMC (1995) state in clauses 28–29 of their guidance for doctors:

'Delegating care to non-medical staff and students:

28. You may delegate medical care to nurses and other health care staff who are not registered medical practitioners if you believe it is best for the patient. But you must be sure that the person to whom you delegate is competent to undertake the procedure or therapy involved. When delegating care or treatment, you must always pass on enough information about the patient and the treatment needed. You will still be responsible for managing the patient's care.

29. You must not enable anyone who is not registered with the GMC to carry out tasks that require the knowledge and skills of a doctor.'

The Joint Consultants Committee (JCC) of the BMA (1996) guidelines is forceful in its advice:

'The JCC believes that all health care professionals should devote their professional time to those tasks that are appropriate for the training that they have received...

Whatever the level of complexity of the task, the doctor responsible for delegating the task and the health care professional responsible for performing the task should always take account of a number of issues...

The name of the general practitioner or hospital consultant holding ultimate clinical responsibility should be known to the patient and all members of the health care team. The doctor will be responsible for any decision to delegate responsibility.

The health care professional to whom the clinical task is to be delegated must have received the appropriate training to be able to perform the task. S/he must be able to recognise complications and know to whom to report should problems occur.

Protocols describing and limiting the task to be performed must be produced. The degree of supervision should be described within the protocol. There should be regular audit of task performance and outcome.

The status of the person performing the procedure must be clearly apparent to the patient; the patient's consent must be obtained before a non-medically qualified health care professional performs a clinical task that has been delegated by a doctor.'

There does need to be some consensus developed between the medical and nursing professions on these issues with ideally a joint statement being produced. Some commonality of approach must be achievable in order to take account of the problems that have been discussed, which clearly affect both doctors and nurses. Darley (1996) suggests a number of ways forward which include:

'... the language used in describing the delegation of tasks from one professional group to another conveys implicit messages of hierarchy and rank. It would be better to talk of referral or "sharing of care".'

Other changes and strategies can be considered but the fundamental message must be as Darley (1996) states:

'The complexity of modern care is such that no single profession can reasonably assume accountability or management responsibility for all care.'

Keeping up to date

Nurses are under a professional duty to keep up to date (UKCC, 1992a,b, 1996). The law also imposes a legal duty, which makes sense as people approach professionals for professional advice and it is implicit in that relationship that up to date information will be given or acted on and that harm maybe suffered if it is not right.

The application of this principle is problematic and will depend on the circumstances of each case. To put into effect what somebody states in a journal could well be negligent if the evidence they have used is faulty and the nurse blindly applies it and injury results. It is the responsibility of the individual nurse making use of the information to properly apply it. Reflective practice is safe practice and the information given must be properly assessed and evidenced-based.

The issue of keeping up to date was considered in *Gascoine* v. *Ian Sheridan and Co (a firm) and Latham* [1994] 5 Med LR 437. An issue in the case concerned the duty of a consultant gynaecologist to keep up to date. Mr Justice Mitchell stated that the ordinary gynaecologists – the judge used the term 'shop floor gynaecologists' – were very busy people who had a responsibility to keep themselves generally informed on mainstream changes in diagnosis, treatment and practice through the mainstream literature such as the leading textbooks and *The Journal of Obstetrics and Gynaecology*. It would, however, be unreasonable to expect them to acquaint themselves with the content of the more obscure journals.

Keeping up to date is a fundamental prerequisite to safe clinical practice. Where nurses are practising at specialist and advanced levels, working in a speciality and performing some medical activities, it will not be unreasonable to expect them to read some of the literature doctors read as well as nursing texts.

Individual accountability

Nurses are individually professionally and legally accountable for their actions and omissions. While the principle of vicarious liability in tort law makes the employer jointly and severally liable along with the nurse for the nurse's negligence, the nurse could still be sued. The principle provides plaintiffs with a financial pocket for damages and operates only where the nurse is an employee and was acting in the course of his or her employment at the time of the negligence. The principle should not detract from the individual professional and legal accountabilities that the nurse maintains.

The negligent nurse would still be in breach of his or her contract of employment and there is also the possibility of an appearance before an internal disciplinary hearing or a UKCC professional conduct committee.

Conclusion

This chapter has hopefully shown that the law relates directly to the specialist and advanced nurse practitioner and to all other nurses and health carers. Patients can be seen to be more litigious and are making more complaints; high litigation and complaint levels have been identified. Patients' motives are various and may be directed to achieve financial compensation for negligence, but it has been seen that often communication problems lie at the core of complaints and cases.

Good patient communication and record keeping strategies are essential to avoid litigation and to effectively manage clinical risk. These strategies also form an essential part of patient advocacy. To be an effective patient advocate nurses must keep good records and communicate properly. It has been seen that the tort of negligence applies to all professionals and the specialist and advanced practitioners can be subject to medical standards of care and skill. All professionals are under a legal duty to keep up to date.

Guidelines from the professional bodies which deal with expanded role issues have been discussed and the conclusion advanced that changes are needed in order to reflect some consensus about expanded role activities. The individual professional and legal accountability of the nurse has also been stressed.

References

Audit Commission (1992) *Making Time for Patients: A Handbook for Ward Sisters.* HMSO, London.

Audit Commission (1993) *What Seems to be the Matter: Communication Between Hospitals and Patients.* HMSO, London.

Audit Commission (1995) *Setting the Records Straight: A Study of Hospital Medical Records.* HMSO, London.

AVMA (1995) *Medical Accidents.* Action for Victims of Medical Accidents, London.

BMA (1996) *Protecting Patient Safety: Medical Procedures Performed by Non-medically Qualified Health Professionals.* Joint Consultants Committee, British Medical Association, London.

CNST (1996) *Risk Management Standards and Procedures: Manual of Guidance*. Clinical Negligence Scheme for Trusts, Bristol.

Darley, M. (1996) Right for the job. *Nursing Times*, **92** (30), 28.

Dowling, S., Martin, R. and Skidmore, P. (1996) Nurses taking on junior doctors' work: a confusion of accountability. *British Medical Journal*, **312**, 1211.

DoH (1994) *Being Heard*. The report of a review committee on NHS complaints procedures. DoH, London.

GMC (1995) *Duties of a Doctor, Good Medical Practice*. General Medical Council, London.

Goodwin, H. & Moss, J. (1997) Clinical risk in A & E nursing. *MDU Nurse*, **8**, 4.

Green, S., Goodwin, H. & Moss, J. (1996) *Problems in General Practice: Complaints and How to Avoid Them*. Medical Defence Union, London.

HSC (1997–8) Health Service Commissioner, first report for session 1997–8. Annual Report for 1996–7. HMSO, London.

Hughes, M. (1996) Key issues in the introduction of nurse endoscopy. *Nursing Times*, **92** (8), 38–9.

Jones, M.A. (1996) *Medical Negligence*, 2nd edn. Sweet and Maxwell, London.

NHS Executive (1996a) *Clinical Negligence and Personal Injury Litigation: Claims Handling*, Executive Letter EL (96) 11. DoH, Leeds.

NHS Executive (1996b) *Clinical Negligence Costs*, Finance Directorate Letter, FDL (96) 39. DoH, Leeds.

NHS Executive (1996c) *Complaints: Listening... Acting... Improving: Guidance on Implementation of the NHS Complaints Procedure*. NHS Executive, Leeds.

Nursing Standard (1996) More responsibility risks legal action. News item. *Nursing Standard*, 30 October, 9.

Nursing Standard (1997) Government orders review of record keeping by nurses. *Nursing Standard*, **11** (46), 5.

Pincombe, C. (1996) CNST: New Standards. *Health Care Risk Report*, **2** (5), 5, 7.

Royal College of Physicians (1997) *Improving communications between doctors and patients*. A report of a working party. Royal College of Physicians of London.

UKCC (1992a) *The Scope of Professional Practice*. UKCC, London.

UKCC (1992b) *Code of Professional Conduct*, 3rd edn. UKCC, London.

UKCC (1993) *Standards for Records and Record Keeping*. UKCC, London.

UKCC (1996) *Guidelines for Professional Practice*. UKCC, London.

Vincent, C., Young, M. & Phillips, A. (1994) Why do people sue doctors? A study of patients and relatives taking legal action. *Lancet*, **343**, 25 June, 1609–13.

Waters, J. (1996) Horror stories warn of need for training. *Nursing Times*, **92** (16), 9.

Chapter 5

Specialist and Advanced Practice: Issues for Research

Paula McGee

Introduction

Castledine's research (Castledine, 1982) was the first to examine the specialist nursing role in England and Wales. His study included both nurses who regarded themselves as what were then called clinical nurse specialists and others whom managers regarded as fulfilling the demands of the role. His results identified 60 different nursing specialties and 353 nurses who held the title of clinical nurse specialist. He compared their work with the criteria for the clinical nurse specialist role which was adopted by the American Nurses Association in 1980 and concluded that only 8% of the UK sample matched these. This study was the first to examine specialist practice in the UK and the only major study in this field until 1996 (McGee *et al.*, 1996).

The amount of British based research is still small and this chapter explores some of the topic areas which require investigation. The author is particularly indebted to the work of Pearson who produces an annual report in the USA on issues to do with advanced practice (Pearson, 1997). Every year Pearson documents the changes made in each state with regard to legal authority, payment and prescribing authority for advanced practitioners. Overall these reports reveal a growing trend in autonomous practice but demonstrate the differences between each state. It is hoped that the programme of research developing at the University of Central England will provide a similar British report, documenting the development of specialist and advanced practice throughout the UK.

Employment conditions

McGee *et al.* (1996) conducted a survey of all the NHS trusts in England following publication of the UKCC's standards for post-registration education and practice (UKCC, 1995). This showed that 58% of trusts employed ten or more specialist nurses and only four had none at all. For advanced practitioners the situation was reversed. Also, 52% of Trusts did not employ advanced practitioners at all and those which did had only one or two. The majority of nurses in both categories were paid at H, G or I grades but the research identified 49 specialist practitioners and 13 advanced practitioners paid at E grade. Five specialist nurses were paid at D grade. There appeared to be no strategy for determining the grading of posts. The majority were considered by the Trusts to be unique in some way and consequently few were able to provide standard job descriptions. While posts may be unique, there must also be commonalities if the nurses concerned are to be recognized as specialist or advanced practitioners by the UKCC. These commonalities should be made explicit so that the whole organization is clear about these forms of practice for the benefit of all. At present it would appear that posts are developed in a fragmentary way, that Trusts do not have policies about specialist and advanced roles which apply across the whole organization.

Consequently each post develops to meet the needs of a specific unit of management. This may be desirable locally but leads to discrepancies throughout the organization and raises additional possibilities. For example, a career as a specialist nurse in stoma care may be more lucrative than one in tissue viability. In addition, since grading is often linked to status, postholders who occupy inferior positions may not have sufficient authority to function. Thus one advanced practitioner in a Trust may have more power than another simply because of the way in which they are perceived. As Castledine (1982) points out, status is an important element in ensuring that the practitioner is taken seriously, not only by other nurses but by colleagues from other professions. Research is therefore needed to examine the rationale for employing specialist and advanced practitioners and the grading of their posts.

Pearson (1997) raises different issues about employment. Advanced nurses in the USA are allowed, under federal legislation, to bill Medicaid and insurance companies as independent practitioners (Doyle, 1991). Arrangements about this vary from state to state. In some the payment is made to the employing organization and in others to the nurse direct. The amount varies but it is usually a percentage of a doctor's fee (Pearson, 1996; Doyle, 1991). It would seem therefore that, in at least some states, nurses are regarded as legitimate providers of services in their own right rather than an adjunct of medicine. In the UK, nurses must market their specialist and advanced skills to convince purchasers in the NHS and insurance companies in the independent sector that they are capable of this type of practice. As Cheshire (1992) has pointed out, this is not an easy option. Her move to becoming a self-employed stoma care nurse highlighted the need for good business and administration skills in order to provide a cost effective service which was also good value for money. If British nurses are to develop in this way, research is needed to identify markets for their skills as well as their associated educational requirements.

Scope of practice

McGee *et al.* (1996) found that specialist nurses were employed in 320 specialties with the most common fields being diabetes, Macmillan nursing, continence advice, infection control and stoma care. Their scope of practice had changed considerably since Castledine's survey (1982) in that most of the Trusts described work roles which, on analysis, conformed to the American criteria for specialist nurses. Thus they had a role in direct patient care, teaching patients, staff and carers, acting as consultant to the Trust and to staff, providing leadership and management plus engaging in research activities (Girard, 1987). Further research is needed to clarify whether practitioners themselves experience their roles in this way, although evidence presented elsewhere in this book would suggest that they do.

McGee *et al.* (1996) found that advanced nurses were employed mainly in accident and emergency, night duty, paediatrics and orthopaedics. In contrast to the specialist practitioners, advanced nurses' roles were less well defined although they were thought to have roles which included clinical practice, research, teaching, practice development, prescribing and even replacing doctors. These findings indicate some confusion about advanced practice and in particular a lack of differentiation between this and the specialist role. It may also reflect a feeling that advanced practice was imposed from the top down by the UKCC. In contrast with specialist practice, advanced nursing was not seen to have evolved and consequently Trusts did not feel confident that they knew what advanced practice was. There were, however, nurse practitioner roles which were well established in places such as accident and emergency departments and it is possible that some Trusts were also not clear about whether emergency nurse practitioners were the same as advanced nurses. The survey by Kendall *et al.* (1997) would suggest that there are differences between nurse practitioners and advanced nursing but this requires further investigation. Evidence presented in Part 2 of this book suggests that the advanced role is changing and evolving but further research is needed to monitor the development of advanced practice roles. In particular there is a need to clarify the experiences of advanced practitioners themselves as part of establishing a baseline for this form of practice.

Research by McGee *et al.* (1996) raises concerns about the fields of practice in which specialist and advanced nurses are employed. The apparent emphasis on acute adult care needs further investigation; mental health and learning disabilities were significantly under-represented in the results. There may in fact be a lack of specialist and advanced practitioners in these fields but, alternatively, there may be differing interpretations of the roles. Community psychiatric nurses might, for example, be regarded as specialist practitioners within mental health but they may not regard themselves as such unless they have specialized within their field.

In the USA, each state has made different arrangements regarding the scope of advanced practice. The term incorporates those working as clinical nurse-midwives, nurse practitioners, advanced nurse practitioners, clinical nurse anaesthetists and some mental health practitioners. Clinical nurse specialists will also be included in some states from 1998 (Pearson, 1997). This plethora of titles is very confusing and it is difficult at times to determine how far these roles resemble those found in the UK. The situation also raises issues for British nursing about the desirability of new job titles. A few titles which are understood by the majority might be more appropriate.

Each American state has its own laws and state boards for nursing. These are moving gradually towards 'greater authority and autonomy' and none has moved to become more restrictive (Pearson, 1995). In 1997, 26 states recognized the title of advanced practice nurse and practice was governed by the Board of Nursing. A further 16 states stipulated the additional requirement of supervision by a doctor. In six states the title of advanced practice nurse was protected and practice was governed by the Board of Nursing and the Board of Medicine. Only three states had no separate legislation for advanced practice nurses and relied solely on their Nurse Practice Acts (Pearson, 1997). The scope of practice therefore varies from state to state and there are changes every year (see for example Pearson 1995, 1996, 1997).

One of the major differences between the American scope of practice and that of the UK is in prescribing. In 1997, 19 states allowed the advanced practice nurse 'complete and independent authority to prescribe, including controlled substances' without physician involvement. However, two states allowed this only in clearly specified circumstances. Eighteen states allowed the advanced practice nurse to prescribe, including controlled substances, with some degree of supervision by doctors, but three states allowed this only in clearly specified circumstances. Thirteen states allowed the advanced practice nurse to prescribe, excluding controlled substances, with some degree of supervision by a doctor. Fourteen states allowed the advanced practice nurse to dispense medication. Only one state did not allow advanced practice nurses any prescribing authority (Pearson, 1997).

The ability and authority to prescribe depends on a sound education in pharmacology, which has been noticeably absent in nurse education in the UK until quite recently, plus medical co-operation. It requires careful consideration of what the nurse may safely prescribe and in what circumstances. Factors which necessitate referral to a doctor must be clearly stated. Shay *et al.* (1996) recommend the construction of a contract setting out which services will be provided by the nurse and those to be the province of the doctor. Specialist and advanced nurses in the UK may find it useful to explore the possibilities of developing such contracts. At present many of these nurses know exactly what is required but are unable to provide it themselves. For example, a nurse working in the community may be more knowledgeable than the general practitioner about the type of wound dressing a patient requires. Nevertheless, it is only the doctor who is allowed to prescribe the dressing and not the nurse. Such situations are farcical and perpetuate outmoded game playing (Stein, 1967; Stein *et al.*, 1990), which has no place in a professional working relationship based on equality.

Evaluation of the roles

Little attention has been paid in the UK to the evaluation of specialist or advanced nursing posts. For the most part, Trusts have relied on patient satisfaction surveys although some have also used clinical audits and individual performance review (McGee *et al.*, 1996). Patient satisfaction is still a crude evaluative mechanism. Patients may say that they are satisfied but there can be discrepancies between what they are satisfied with and the perceptions of the health care providers (Donabedian, 1960). Thus a patient may state that they are satisfied with the care received when they actually meant, 'Thank goodness I survived, in spite of what the professionals did!' Patients may also fear reprisals if they seem less than grateful (Koch, 1994). This is not to say that patients do not have the right to express their views or that their opinions are invalid, but that patient satisfaction should be used in conjunction with other methods of evaluation. Patients may state that they like a particular specialist nurse, even value that nurse's contribution to their care, but that does not mean patients understand what a specialist or advanced practitioner is. Nor does it give managers insight into the cost effectiveness of that care, how it differs from that provided by other nurses or the ways in which the postholder functions. Research is therefore needed to determine:

- How patients experience care provided by specialist and advanced nurses and how this differs from that given by professional practitioners.
- The most appropriate tools for evaluating the effectiveness of specialist and advanced practice both within specific specialities and across organizations.

Conclusion

This chapter has explored some of the possible avenues for investigation into specialist and advanced nursing practice in the UK. In some instances these have been compared to developments in North America. This is not to imply that British nursing should adopt wholesale the strategies used in another country. The emphasis is on providing ideas and raising awareness of issues which have arisen elsewhere and which should be addressed, even if they are to be discarded. It is hoped that the next 10 years will see a steady growth in research into specialist and advanced practice and that the development of each is well documented.

References

Castledine, G. (1982) The role and function of clinical nurse specialists in England and Wales. Unpublished MSc dissertation, University of Manchester.

Cheshire, L. (1992) An independent stoma care service. *Nursing Times*, 9 September, (51), 28–30.

Donabedian, A. (1960) The definitions of quality and approaches to its assessment. *Explorations in Quality and Monitoring*, vol. 1. Health Administration Press, Ann Arbor.

Doyle, E. (1991) Third party reimbursement – advanced nursing practice. *The Missouri Nurse*, **60** (3), 12–13.

Girard, N. (1987) The CNS: development of the role. In: *The Clinical Nurse Specialist: Perspectives on Practice* (ed. S. Menard). John Wiley and Sons, New York.

Kendall, S., Latter, S. & Ryecroft-Malone, J. (1997) *Nursing's hand in the new deal. Nurse practitioners and secondary health care in North Thames.* Buckinghamshire College, Chalfont St Giles.

Koch, T. (1994) Establishing rigour in qualitative research: the decision trail. *Journal of Advanced Nursing*, **19**, 976–86.

McGee, P., Castledine, G. & Brown, R. (1996) *A survey of specialist and advanced nursing practice in England.* Research report published by the Nursing Research Unit, University of Central England, Birmingham.

Pearson, L. (1995) Annual update of how each state stands on legislative issues affecting advanced nursing practice. *Nurse Practitioner*, **20** (1).

Pearson, L. (1996) Annual update of how each state stands on legislative issues affecting advanced nursing practice. *Nurse Practitioner*, **21** (1).

Pearson, L. (1997) Annual update of how each state stands on legislative issues affecting advanced nursing practice. *Nurse Practitioner*, **22** (1).

Shay, L., Goldstein, J., Matthews, D., Trail, L. & Edmunds, M. (1996) Guidelines for developing a nurse practitioner practice. *Nurse Practitioner*, **21** (1), 72–81.

Stein, P. (1967) The doctor–nurse game. *Archives of General Psychiatry*, 3 (27), 993–5.

Stein, P., Watts, D. & Howell, T. (1990) The doctor–nurse game revisited. *New England Journal of Medicine*, **322** (8), 546–9.

UKCC (1995) *PREP and You.* United Kingdom Central Council for Nursing, Midwifery and Health Visiting, London.

Chapter 6

Advanced Physical Assessment

*Susan Cohen, Patricia Polgar Bailey,
Clarice Begemann and Kate Moffett*

The process of physical assessment or health assessment resembles a mystery story or puzzle. The health care provider uses many avenues to elicit clues and cues to understanding a patient's general health status as well as any acute or chronic health problems. Health assessment provides the initial information from the patient and adds to the ability to care for patients over time. The tools or skills needed to navigate the assessment maze are active listening, comprehensive history taking, keen visual observation and the learned manoeuvres of physical examination.

Advanced practice nurses (APNs) use health assessment as part of the continuous process of caring for patients. Numerous guides to health assessment are available in books, videotapes and educational programmes. However, the process of assessment includes both the skills in eliciting information and the decision making process regarding the information gained through health assessment. Brykczynski (1985) identified management of patient health/illness in ambulatory care settings as one of the domains of advanced practice nursing. This area of skilled practice encompasses:

(1) Assessing, monitoring, co-ordinating and managing the health status of patients over time
(2) Detecting acute and chronic disease
(3) Providing anticipatory guidance for changes
(4) Building and maintaining a supportive and caring attitude
(5) Scheduling follow-up visits to monitor patients closely in uncertain situations
(6) Selecting and recommending appropriate diagnostic and therapeutic interventions and regimes.

To illustrate the process of health assessment and management, three case studies are presented. The individuals in the case studies all have a chronic illness with the complexity of psychosocial and cultural factors impacting which affect their health. The three case studies represent 'real life' clinical situations with significant personal details altered to prevent identification of any particular patient. Each case demonstrates a slightly different approach to the assessment process. The first case of a patient with hypertension follows the APN's actions and decisions in a narrative format. The second case presents quick glimpses of the APN's decision-making through reflection of the process. The final case demonstrates decision-making in a series of questions or considerations within the ongoing assessment. The cases are presented with assessed patient data and the decision-making process of the APN to illuminate the discovery and management process of health assessment.

Case study – hypertension

The following case focuses on a 47-year-old male, Mr X, who has hypertension. Mr X receives his health care at a clinic affiliated with a local hospital. Mr X was initially referred to the clinic two years ago by the occupational nurse at his place of employment. His blood pressure on three separate occasions at work was noted to be 170/100–180/100 mmHg. He denied a previous diagnosis of high blood pressure but also could not remember the last time that it was checked. The occupational health nurse, appropriately concerned about these persistent elevations in blood pressure, referred the patient to the clinic, at which time he was completely asymptomatic. The discussion includes a summary of the events and clinical decisions surrounding Mr X's initial appointment, diagnosis and subsequent clinical course.

At the clinic he was seen by an APN for the evaluation and management of possible hypertension. After introducing herself to the patient, the APN interviews him to obtain a health history. In addition to getting to know the patient, she also wants to determine whether Mr X's hypertension is primary or secondary (JNC, 1993). The other aims of a thorough history and physical examination are to assess whether hypertension has caused any tissue or organ damage, to detect lifestyle habits which may be contributing to the hypertension, and to identify the presence of other factors which increase Mr X's risk for cardiovascular disease.

Mr X's past medical history was significant only for obesity (height 5 ft 10 in; weight 230 lb). Mr X denied taking any medications including over-the-counter preparations. He works full-time in a state agency and is engaged to be married in several months. He has smoked 1–2 packs of cigarettes per day for the last 15 years. He limits his alcohol intake to a couple of beers on Friday and Saturday evenings. He denies a problem with alcoholism or any illicit drug use. He follows no specific diet and enjoys a lot of fatty and salty foods. He drinks 1–2 cups of coffee as well as several caffeinated sodas throughout the course of the day. Mr X denies getting any regular exercise.

Mr X's family history is significant for a father who died in his early sixties of a heart attack. His paternal grandmother died of diabetes-related complications. His sisters has hypertension.

Table 6.1 shows key components of the medical history.

Table 6.1   Key components of the medical history.

(1)	Information on previous blood pressure values and the duration and severity of known hypertension
(2)	Effectiveness and side effects of any prior antihypertensive medications
(3)	Symptoms that may be due to secondary cause of hypertension
(4)	Symptoms suggestive of heart, nervous system or kidney disease
(5)	Usual or recent weight and any weight changes over the past years
(6)	History of diabetes, cigarette smoking, exercise habits, and cholesterol (total, HDL (high density lipoprotein), LDL (low density lipoprotein), triglycerides)
(7)	Dietary habits including intake of sodium, cholesterol and saturated fats
(8)	Alcohol use
(9)	Information on domestic and work-related environments
(10)	Medication use (prescription and over-the-counter)
(11)	Family history including hypertension, premature coronary heart disease, stroke, diabetes and hyperlipidemia (Margolis & Klag, 1996)

After obtaining a careful health history, the APN begins the physical examination. Mr X is observed to be a mildly obese gentleman in no distress. Physical examination results from this encounter are represented in Table 6.2.

On this initial visit to the clinic, Mr X is diagnosed with Stage II (moderate) hypertension (JNC, 1993). In addition, the APN is concerned about several other factors which could be contributing to Mr X's hypertension, as well as risk for cardiovascular disease. He is obese which affects blood pressure by increasing peripheral resistance. Also, he admits to excess sodium intake which also increases blood pressure by increasing total fluid volume and preload. Other cardiovascular risk factors include smoking, male gender and a familial history of cardiac disease (Margolis & Klag, 1996).

Essential v. secondary hypertension

Around 90–95% of patients aged 18–65 will have no identifiable cause for their hypertension (Margolis & Klag, 1996). This is called essential or primary hypertension. However, hypertension does not exist in every

Table 6.2 Mr X's physical examination.

Vital signs	Apical pulse 78, respiratory rate 18, blood pressure 170/100
Head, eyes, ears, neck and throat	Pupils equal and reactive to light, discs sharp, fundi without exudates, without haemorrhages, no AV nicking Extraocular movements intact, visual acuity 20/25 bilaterally without correction, no icterus Neck supple, no adenopathy, no thyroid enlargement
Respiratory	Clear to auscultation bilaterally, full inspiration bilaterally
Cardiac	Normal S1, S2, regular rate and rhythm, no murmurs
Abdomen	Mildly protuberant, normal bowel sounds in all quadrants, soft, non-tender, no masses or organomegaly
Rectal	Good rectal tone, no masses, stool sample for occult blood – negative
Musculoskeletal	Full range of motion all extremities without pain or crepitus. 5/5 strength bilaterally
Vascular	Upper and lower extremities, no cyanosis, clubbing or oedema
Neurological	Alert and oriented × 3, cranial nerves II-XII intact, 2/2 deep tendon reflexes bilaterally, gait normal

society. There are environmental or lifestyle factors, such as eating habits, activity and possible stress, which may play a role in the development of hypertension (JNC, 1993).

Studies of twins and family members indicate that there may be a genetic component in essential hypertension (Margolis & Klag, 1996). Research suggests that the implicated gene is one that controls the body's production and release of angiotensinogen. This substance is converted in the bloodstream to angiotension II, a potent vasoconstrictor. Hypertension is also related to an increase in body water and sodium. Increased sodium and water retention increases fluid volume which increases preload and ultimately cardiac output. However, the underlying basis for sodium and water retention is not known. Genetic alteration and excess sodium intake may play a role. Stress may play a role in hypertension. Stress induces sympathetic nervous system overactivity which increases cardiac contractility and ultimately increases cardiac output.

Hypertension in which there is an identifiable cause is called secondary hypertension. Although secondary hypertension is a much less common

Table 6.3 Secondary causes of hypertension.

The most common causes of secondary hypertension include:

- Drugs such as corticosteroids, cold remedies, nasal decongestants, appetite suppressants, cyclosporine, erythropoietin, MAO inhibitors, tricyclic antidepressants, cocaine, amphetamines and non-steroidal anti-inflammatory drugs. Hypertension due to drug use is usually transient; blood pressure should return to normal within a few weeks of discontinuation of the drug.
- Kidney disease, especially that leading to chronic renal failure, almost always produces hypertension.
- Adrenal tumours including primary aldosteronism, Cushing's syndrome, and pheochromocytoma.
- Other hormonal causes such as hyperthyroidism, hypothyroidism, excess growth hormone released by a pituitary tumour, or increased blood calcium levels associated with a parathyroid gland tumour.
- Coarctation of the aorta or a constriction of a portion of the aorta in the chest; clues are a decreased blood pressure in the lower extremities and a high blood pressure in the upper extremities.
- Chronic alcoholism over a sustained period of time causes hypertension in some individuals.

type of hypertension, underlying causes should be considered as possible aetiology until ruled out. Table 6.3 shows the most common causes of secondary hypertension.

Information obtained from the health history, at the initial physical examination or during follow-up, will identify those patients who may have hypertension due to an underlying cause. In most cases the work-up to rule out secondary causes can be done without costly evaluations. Clues of possible secondary causes from the history and physical examination (Table 6.4) include a thorough drug history including prescribed, over-the-counter and illicit drug use.

In addition to the history and physical examination, the APN orders some laboratory tests and diagnostic procedures. Laboratory tests she orders include a urinalysis, complete blood count (CBC), sodium (Na), potassium (K), calcium (Ca), creatinine, glucose, uric acid values and a lipid profile. In addition, an electrocardiogram (ECG) is obtained. These laboratory tests are done for several reasons which include:

(1) To help rule out secondary causes as well as establish treatable aetiology
(2) To assess for end organ damage
(3) To establish baseline data so as to treat the patient effectively
(4) To guide the selection of initial treatment
(5) To establish pretreatment status that might be affected by drug therapy and to assess for additional cardiovascular risk factors.

Table 6.4   Clues from the history and physical examination of possible secondary causes of hypertension.

Drugs
A thorough drug history including prescribed, over-the-counter and illicit drug use.

Kidney disease
Renovascular disease is suggested by findings which include:
(1)   the presence of a unilateral high-pitched abdominal bruit radiating to the flank
(2)   well-documented recent (1–2 yr) change from normal BP to Stage II or II hypertension
(3)   hypertension refractory to maximally tolerated doses of multiple antihypertensive drugs
(4)   unexplained refractoriness to previously effective drugs
(5)   a very high baseline diastolic pressure (e.g. 115 mm Hg) in a person less than 30 years of age
(6)   evidence of accelerated hypertension (i.e. Stage III or IV, retinopathy, renal insufficiency due to hypertension) in any patient

Kidney disease should be suspected as a possible cause in:
(1)   hypertensive patients with a history of haematuria, stones and recurrent pyelonephritis
(2)   patients in whom large kidneys (e.g. due to obstruction or polycystic kidney disease) or a large bladder (after voiding) are palpated
(3)   when urinalysis suggests acute or chronic glomerulonephritis (i.e. proteinuria and/or many casts, especially red cell casts)

Adrenal tumours
Primary hyperaldosteronism is caused by excess secretion of aldosterone (not caused by angiotensin II stimulation) by the adrenal cortex. The most common clue is a baseline potassium significantly below normal for which there is no explanation. Hypertensive patients with this finding should be questioned about excess liquorice consumption which contains an ingredient with mineral cortocoid-like activity.

Cushing's syndrome which involves another adrenal cortex tumour that secretes excessive amounts of cortisone, and related tumours. Clues include pheochromocytoma which is caused by excess release of epinephrine and nor-epinephrine by tumours of the central or medullary portion of the adrenal gland. Clues are a history of a hypermetabolic state and/or paroxysms of symptoms caused by increased sympathetic nervous system activity (tachycardia, palpitations, diaphoresis) with associated severe headaches. The absence of such a cluster of symptoms viritually excludes the presence of a pheochromocytoma.

Other hormonal causes may be considered further if clinical examination and laboratory work suggests thyroid disease, parathyroid or pituitary tumours.

Coarctation of the aorta is suggested by:
(1)   hyertension in a relatively young patient
(2)   decreased blood pressure in the lower extremities
(3)   evidence of collateral arterial circulation on inspection of the trunk or on chest X-ray which may also show post-stenotic dilatation of the aorta

Chronic alcoholism as determined by a careful health history or suggested by behaviour patterns.

For example, the APN is aware that an elevated serum creatinine or protein in the urine is probable evidence of kidney disease, and a low potassium should raise her suspicion of adrenal disorders such as primary hyper-aldosteronism and Cushing's syndrome. She knows that a fasting glucose and lipid profile will be helpful in determining whether the patient has diabetes or lipid abnormalities, which in addition to contributing to his risk for cardiovascular disease would guide decision-making regarding phar-macological therapy if and when that is indicated. Table 6.5 shows the laboratory findings.

Table 6.5   Mr X's laboratory findings.

Urinalysis	Within normal limits
Labs	Complete blood count – within normal limits Sodium – within normal limits Potassium – within normal limits Calcium – within normal limits Creatinine – within normal limits Glucose – within normal limits Uric acid – within normal limits
Lipid profile	Total cholesterol – 210 High density lipoprotein – 35 Low density lipoprotein – 165 Triglycerides – 190
Electrocardiogram	Normal sinus rhythm, no ectopy, no evidence of ischaemia or infarction, no evidence of left ventricular hypertrophy

Based on his history, physical and laboratory/diagnostic evaluation, the APN concludes that Mr X has Stage II (moderate) hypertension. His work-up does not suggest other underlying aetiology, nor does it appear that Mr X has suffered tissue or end-organ damage as a result of previous undiagnosed or untreated hypertension.

In addition to hypertension, Mr X has several other co-existing cardio-vascular risk factors including obesity, hyperlipidemia, smoking, a rela-tively sedentary lifestyle, his gender and a familial history of cardiovascular disease. Since sustained high blood pressure had been confirmed, one of the nurse practitioner's goals at this point was to help Mr X restore his blood pressure to normal, thereby reducing his risk of future cardiovascular disease. In addition, as part of the treatment of any hypertensive patient, a second goal is the control or reduction of as many of his other alterable cardiovascular risk factors as possible.

Since Mr X does not have accelerated hypertension, malignant hyper-tension or hypertensive urgency, the first step in trying to lower his blood pressure is with lifestyle modification.

Table 6.6 Diagnosis and classifications of blood pressure (JNC, 1993).

Category	Systolic BP (mmHg)	Diastolic BP (mmHg)
Normal	< 130	< 85
High normal	130–139	85–89
Hypertension		
Stage I (mild)	140–159	90–99
Stage II (moderate)	160–179	100–109
Stage III (severe)	180–209	110–119
Stage IV (very severe)	> 210	> 120

In accelerated hypertension, there is clinical evidence of severe arterio-sclerosis, meaning either grade 3 or 4 retinopathy, or renal insufficiency of which there is no apparent cause except the hypertension. Before developing evidence of accelerated hypertension, most of these patients have had very high blood pressure for one or more years. The prognosis in untreated accelerated hypertension is poor: approximately 95% of patients die of cardiac, renal or CNS complications within five years of initial presentation. Control of blood pressure, even in those patients with end stage renal disease, can dramatically improve the prognosis.

In malignant hypertension, severe elevation of blood pressure will predictably cause a catastrophic outcome within hours or days, e.g. hypertensive encephalopathy and dissecting aneurysm of the thoracic aorta. This is a hypertensive emergency. Should such patients present in the office setting, they need to be transported to an emergency facility.

Hypertensive urgency is used to categorize patients with severe hypertension (systolic blood pressure >210 mmHg and/or diastolic blood pressure >120 mmHg) who are asymptomatic.

The APN discusses with Mr X his diagnosis of hypertension as well as why control of blood pressure is so important. She understands that for many asymptomatic individuals the importance of blood pressure control is difficult to understand since, like Mr X, they feel well. She talks with Mr X about the effects of sustained high blood pressure on other organs like the kidneys and also the risk of high blood pressure for other cardiovascular problems like heart disease. She talks with Mr X about his father's heart disease and the fact that blood pressure control will decrease the risk of him suffering a heart attack. She also discusses the importance of reducing some of his other cardiovascular risk factors such as his elevated cholesterol, obesity and smoking. They discuss the fact that certain risks such as his familial history and his gender are unalterable, that he has no control over these. She emphasizes that the risk factors that are alterable, such as his blood pressure, weight, lifestyle, alcohol and smoking, are things to work on. They also discuss the effect of chronic alcohol use on blood pressure. She talks with Mr X about the possible need for an alcohol detoxification programme but he assures her that this will not be necessary.

The APN and Mr X agree that he will work on several of the most important issues which he feels are feasible. Mr X agrees to try and make some modifications in his diet, specifically decreasing the amount of fatty and fried foods and using a salt substitute. In addition, he agrees to try to cut down to one pack per day of cigarettes and decrease his alcohol consumption to two beers per day rather than a case. She discusses smoking cessation strategies with him. They also discuss the role of exercise in reducing blood pressure as well as how to incorporate physical activity on a regular basis. The APN provides Mr X with written information on decreased cholesterol diets and reviews these with him in the office. In addition, she gives him information about local smoking cessation groups. She also reiterates the offer of an outpatient alcohol detoxification programme but Mr X declines her offer. She also gives him patient education literature on hypertension to read at home and they agree to discuss this and any other questions he may have on his return visit.

The APN understands that Mr X has been given a lot of information today – both a diagnosis of hypertension and lots of teaching about blood pressure control. They agree that he will come back in one month and that during the interval he will ask the occupational health nurse to check his blood pressure at least once a week. Mr X agrees to call the APN with his blood pressure readings. She gives Mr X her office number and encourages him to call her should he have any questions, concerns or problems prior to his next visit.

Mr X misses his following appointment in one month despite calls from the nurse practitioner emphasizing the importance of follow-up. He misses two subsequent appointments and finally returns four months later. At this time his blood pressure is 160/100. Mr X had gained 2 lb since his initial visit but otherwise there were no significant changes. He is unclear regarding the reason for his missed appointments.

Mr X reports being successful in decreasing his salt·intake; he now uses a salt substitute and only occasionally adds salt to his food while cooking it. His fiancée is with him during this visit and substantiates this. She appears to be quite concerned about his blood pressure and both he and she agree that she is even more vigilant regarding dietary changes. He has tried to decrease his intake of fried and fatty foods. He states he has cut back 1–2 cigarettes per day.

The APN does a focused physical examination and then discusses her impression with Mr X. She provides positive feedback for the changes he has made, such as decreasing his salt and fat intake. She expresses her concern regarding his persistently elevated blood pressure and discusses the need for initiating pharmacological therapy due to the lack of adequate response to lifestyle modifications during the last four months.

Since it has been four months since Mr X's last visit, the APN would like to check another lipid profile. However, since he is not fasting today, she decides to postpone this until his next visit and discusses with him the need for an early morning appointment in order to get a fasting lipid profile.

The APN is aware of the different antihypertensive drug options available and considers whether to start Mr X on a thiazide diuretic or a beta-blocker antihypertensive medication. The Joint National Commission has recommended diuretics and beta-blockers as initial monotherapy for hypertension. The logic behind this recommendation is that these are the only agents that have been shown in clinical trials to date to reduce morbidity and mortality (JNC, 1993).

Other factors which should be considered in the selection of an antihypertensive agent are demographic characteristics and the existence of other diseases and health problems. For example, in patients with hypertension and congestive heart failure, angiotensin-converting enzyme inhibitors (ACE inhibitors) are considered the drug of choice because they are effective in treating both disease entities (JNC, 1993). Similarly, ACE inhibitors are considered the best antihypertensive agents for diabetic patients with hypertension (Wood, 1996). Alpha-blockers are often used effectively to treat hypertensive patients who suffer from benign prostatic hypertrophy. Patients with hypertension and vasospastic angina generally do well with a calcium channel blocker. These examples illustrate the fact that many antihypertensive agents can be used effectively to treat other health problems in addition to hypertension.

Hypertension is often a syndrome of multiple abnormalities such as hyperlipidemia, diabetes, or left ventricular hypertrophy. To meet the challenge of treating hypertension, the nurse practitioner should select the drug therapy which treats as many of the aspects of the syndrome in addition to lowering the blood pressure. Whenever possible an agent that can treat multiple conditions should be chosen. Conversely, some antihypertensive agents may be relatively or absolutely contraindicated because of coexisting diseases. Some drugs may improve blood pressure control but worsen other diseases. For example, beta-blockers may worsen asthma, diabetes and peripheral ischaemia even though blood pressure is lowered. Whenever possible an agent should be chosen that can effectively treat multiple conditions without worsening others (JNC, 1993).

The APN takes into consideration Mr X's high blood pressure as well as his other health problems. In addition, she considers the side effects of the antihypertensive agents. She knows that beta-blockers tend to have adverse effects on lipid profiles. In addition, she knows that all the thiazide diuretics, with the exception of indapamide, have the potential for worsening existing hyperlipidemia. Furthermore, she knows that there may be population specific differences in the effects of antihypertensive agents on lipids. She is aware that Mr X, depending on his racial or ethnic background, may be more susceptible than patients from other racial and ethnic minority groups to cholesterol increases following diuretic therapy (JNC, 1993).

Of all the thiazide diuretics, indapamide is considered to be lipid neutral and therefore is a good choice for Mr X. However, she has mixed feelings about prescribing this drug for Mr X since it is also significantly more expensive than any of the other thiazide diuretics such as hydrochlorothiazide. The APN checks to see if his insurance will cover his medications. She finds out that it will and is less reluctant to prescribe it. She knows that even if the cost of his care is increased in the short term because of more expensive drug therapy, his long-term medical costs will be less expensive if his risk for cardiovascular disease is decreased by not worsening his hyperlipidemia.

The APN prescribes a low dose of indapamide (2.5 mg/day) for Mr X. She explains the rationale for starting him on pharmacological therapy at this time. Medication teaching includes the side effects of the drug. The APN emphasizes the importance of continuing with non-pharmacological efforts as well, specifically weight reduction, exercise, diet and smoking cessation. She asks Mr X about any concerns or questions he has about the new medication. They agree on a two week follow-up visit to assess the effect of this new medication. The APN encourages Mr X to call her in the interim if he has any concerns about the possible side effects of this medication.

Case study – asymptomatic hypoglycaemia in a patient with non-insulin dependent diabetes mellitus and hypertension

Mrs C, a 78 year old woman with an eight year history of non-insulin dependent diabetes mellitus (NIDDM) and hypertension (HTN), was seen one week ago for a complaint of finger cramping, and has been scheduled today on a Friday afternoon for follow-up of this problem, but the nature of the visit quickly changes when the patient is discovered to be hypoglycaemic.

The triage nurse has taken Mrs C's weight, blood pressure, pulse and random capillary blood glucose, and alerts the nurse practitioner that Mrs C looks great and says she feels fine, but her finger stick glucose is 49. Blood pressure in left arm sitting is 148/88, pulse 84, respirations 20. The APN thanks the triage nurse for being astute and for reporting right away, and requests her to obtain 15 mg of oral glucose and give it to Mrs C immediately. The APN recognizes the urgent need to raise the blood glucose level, and has delegated this responsibility to a nurse so that she can evaluate the patient directly.

Mrs C and her daughter are chatting with each other amicably. The APN asks Mrs C how she feels. Mrs C's response is 'good'. She denies feeling lightheaded, weak, trembling, shaky, sweating, cold or clammy. The APN tells Mrs C that her blood sugar is low, and that she needs some sugar now in order to raise it. The triage nurse enters the room, gives Mrs C the 15 mg of glucose, and will return in 15 minutes to recheck her blood glucose (Rifkin & Porte, 1990).

Mrs C is asked to sit on the examination table. She is a lively, pleasant woman, walks quickly, and rises from sitting to go to the examining table without difficulty, and with good balance. The APN elicits Mrs C's diet history. Breakfast consisted of two pieces of bread and coffee with a teaspoon of real sugar four hours ago, and she had a glass of milk half an hour ago. No lunch on account of her 1 PM appointment here today. The APN again reviews the symptoms of hypoglycaemia in slightly different words, looking for any evidence of sweating, nausea, hunger, lightheadness, palpitations, chest pain, racing heart, changes in vision, difficulty thinking or speaking, headaches, loss of memory, severe decrease in energy, irritability or decreased sensations. Mrs C states she has not experienced any of these symptoms. She has not changed her diet nor her exercise level, did not do any strenuous exercise today, nor does she drink alcohol.

Reassured by Mrs C's answers and behaviour that she is not in any acute distress, the APN proceeds with the history and examination, continually observing the patient for neurological signs of hypoglycaemia such as change in consciousness, coordination, balance or speech. Often patients whose blood glucose levels have been in good control are not symptomatic unless blood glucose levels fall below 40 mg/dl (Speicher, 1993).

Asked again if she ever notes any of these symptoms, Mrs C says she gets a little shaky and nervous feeling maybe twice a week, but a small glass of orange juice takes care of it in a few minutes, and the symptoms are not bothersome. She has noted them for a few months, and cannot recall if they happen at any particular time of day, or when she has not eaten for many hours. She never awakens at night with these symptoms. The nurse practitioner seeks subjective information from the patient regarding hypoglycaemia and possible triggers.

Mrs C's BP and pulse are repeated after she has sat quietly on the examination table for several minutes, and the values are left arm 146/84, pulse 82. The APN is monitoring the cardiovascular system for any signs of increasing hypoglycaemia, such as increasing pulse rate. The APN realizes that the overriding concern from a provider's point of view at the present visit is Mrs C's diabetic control, the present episode of low blood glucose in a non-fasting state, and the probability by history that Mrs C has been experiencing fairly frequent hypoglycaemic episodes. Since the patient's condition is stable, and action has been taken to remedy the low glucose level, the nurse practitioner now feels comfortable to attend to the matter of finger cramping. She gathers the history of her 'cramps' over the intervening week while proceeding with the examination which focuses on the neurological system, looking for evidence of abnormalities that might indicate why Mrs C is having finger cramping. The APN is thus caring for the *patient's* main concern as well as attending to the currently asymptomatic yet hypoglycaemic state.

Mrs C reports that the finger cramps are the same in quality of pain and in duration, and have occurred five of the seven evenings, and that the 'detective' work looking for associations with activity or diet has not revealed any new information. The information the APN gathered from last week's visit for finger cramping is shown in Table 6.7.

The APN has enquired into the seven parameters of pain, and has looked for signs and symptoms of dehydration, hypo- or hyperglycaemia, and

Table 6.7 Analysis of the symptom – finger cramping.

Nature of the problem	New onset of painful involuntary contractures in all her fingers, usually in both hands simultaneously
Quality of pain	'Cramping', sharp
Location of pain	Generalized in the fingers, non radiating
Onset	Two to three weeks ago
Frequency	Once or twice a day
Timing	Evening or before bed, usually three to four hours postprandial
Duration	Less than a minute
Associated symptoms	None; patient feels well when cramps occur; denies numbness, tingling, decreased sensation; denies other cramps elsewhere including large muscle groups including gastrocnemius; denies hypo or hyper glycaemic symptoms; denies change in activity, fluid intake or urinary output; denies feeling overheated or perspiring; no noted heat or cold intolerance, no diarrhoea or constipation, no change in skin moisture, no nervousness or lethargy, no palpitations, no change in appetite or weight, no change in mood
Precipitating events	None identified (no repetitive actions such as knitting, washing, typing, writing)
Relieving factors	Forcibly extending fingers or shaking hands

hypo- or hyperthyroidism, which could be causing muscle cramping. She has also searched for clues of precipitating events such as repetitive actions, which could point towards a neurological source of the cramping (Goroll *et al.*, 1995).

At the last visit the APN had carefully reviewed Mrs C's medicines (Table 6.8) with her, to evaluate proper dosing. Today Mrs C has brought her medicines with her as was requested, and even though the prescription instructions are written in English and her primary language is Spanish, she has written the purpose of the pills on the labels. She correctly identifies the pills by colour and size, giving the correct administration schedule. The number of pills in the bottle and the prescription date also indicate that she is taking the medicines as prescribed. She is not taking any home remedies or botanical preparations.

Table 6.8   Current medications.

For diabetes	Glyburide 10 mg bid (sulphonylurea); Metformin 500 bid (biguanide)
For hypertension	Indapamide 2.5 mg q am (diuretic/vasodilator); Lisinopril 5 mg q am (angiotension converting enzyme inhibitor)

Mrs C reports diabetic medications taken 20 minutes before breakfast and 20 minutes before dinner. Blood pressure medications taken in the morning with her diabetic medications.

The APN has elicited specific information from the patient herself as to how she takes her medicines, and then has validated this information by having the patient demonstrate the pills/uses/etc. She has enquired into alternative therapies.

The APN had developed a differential diagnosis for muscle cramping, considering neurological compromise, dehydration with electrolyte imbalances, hypothyroidism, severe hypoglycaemia, fatiguing exercises, hypocalcaemia and hypomagnesaemia. The APN is also considering ischaemia as a source of pain which could feel like cramps but not be accompanied by contracture (Goroll *et al.*, 1995).

The APN had performed a focused physical examination at the previous visit which revealed no evidence of hypo- or hyperthyroidism, hypo- or hyperglycaemia, dehydration, or neurological or cardiac compromise (Table 6.9). At that point the reason for the cramping was unknown, and the nurse practitioner wanted to rule out electrolyte and elemental imbalances as a source of the cramping, given that Mrs C is taking a diuretic. The plan was for Mrs C to continue to monitor her symptoms, and to play detective to look for any possible trends especially in relation to

Table 6.9 Physical examination from the previous visit.

Vital signs	Height 5 ft 2 in, 158 lb (70 kg), unchanged. Blood pressure, left arm, sitting is 140/88 mmHg.
Laboratory	Random blood glucose capillary finger stick was 95, approximately three hours post-prandial. Urine dipstick revealed pH 6.0, specific gravity of 1.010, trace protein, negative for glucose, negative for ketones, negative for heme.

caloric intake, or precipitating factors such as activity. No changes were made in her medication regimen.

Lab tests were obtained to rule out electrolyte imbalances, hypocalcaemia and hypomagnesaemia. A haemoglobin A1C, which measures fluctuations in blood glucose levels over time, was ordered to gain insight into her diabetic control, as Mrs C does not perform home glucose monitoring. The labs from this previous visit revealed a slightly low magnesium level, and a haemoglobin A1C of 6.1. The reference range for the lab doing the test for non-diabetics is less than 6. This value indicates that her blood glucose ranges have been nearly euglycaemic, and argues against many hyperglycaemic episodes, but may indicate a greater chance of hypoglycaemic episodes (American Diabetes Association, 1997).

Today, the APN repeats the physical examination (Table 6.10). After reassuring Mrs C that her physical examination is normal, the APN begins a conversation about the hypoglycaemic symptoms Mrs C has been having. Mrs C states that she knows this is part of diabetes and the orange juice (approximately 4 ounces) takes care of it, so she has never mentioned it to a provider. The APN teaches the patient about abnormally low blood glucose levels, their symptoms, and praises the patient for taking the correct measures to alleviate the symptoms. The APN explains that changes in Mrs C's diabetic medicines are going to be made to try to find a balance where these symptoms are not occurring, and that if they do she should call and report them. She also explains that Mrs C has taken the right action to alleviate the symptoms of hypoglycaemia, but when diet, exercise and medicines are all in balance, she should not be having these symptoms. Therefore it is important to note and report when they are occurring so that Mrs C and her providers can work together to try to prevent such episodes (Beaser & Hill, 1995). By building on the knowledge Mrs C has, and supporting her correct actions for remedying hypoglycaemia, the nurse practitioner is strengthening Mrs C's knowledge and control of her disease.

The nurse comes in to recheck the capillary blood glucose, which gives the APN a chance to leave the room and assess Mrs C's hypoglycaemia. A quick chart review reveals that Mrs C has had random blood glucose levels of 227, 98 and 85, on approximately monthly intervals over the past three

Table 6.10 Repeat physical examination.

Physical examination	Mrs C is lively, moves easily, responds readily and appropriately.
Skin	Warm, and not dry, normal turgor (no tenting).
Head, eyes, ears, neck and throat	Eyes: pupils equal and reactive to light and accommodation, mucous membranes moist. Neck: supple, no lymphadenopathy, thyroid smooth, non-enlarged, non-tender cervical spine without visible or palpable misalignment, non-tender. Full active range of motion without pain. Keeping the neck in the extreme degrees of range of motion does not cause any tingling, numbness or cramping in her arms or hands.
Cardiac	S1, S2 without additional heart sounds, regular rate and rhythm; radial and pedal pulses within normal limits bilaterally; no carotid bruits.
Muscular-skeletal	Back: trapezius without spasm or tenderness. Upper extremities: symmetric, no atrophy, no hypertrophy. No thenar prominence wasting bilaterally. Full active range of motion in her shoulders, elbows and wrist without pain.
Neurological	Hand grasps are 5/5 bilaterally, sustained flexion of the fingers does not elicit cramping. Deep tendon reflexes of the biceps, triceps, and brachio-radialis are 2+ (normal) and symmetric bilaterally. Dermatomes of the arms and hands bilaterally are intact to sharp point, light touch and vibration. Tinel and phelan tests (to detect carpal tunnel syndrome) are negative bilaterally. No Babinski, negative Romberg (no evidence of central nervous system compromise).

months on random blood glucose tests at the health centre. On none of these visits has Mrs C complained of or responded in the affirmative when asked about symptoms of hypoglycaemia or hyperglycaemia, according to chart notes. Another haemoglobin A1C from three months ago, after being on metformin and glyburide for three months, was 5.9, about the same as that obtained last week, indicating fairly stable blood glucose control; it does not lead one to think that there have been radical changes in Mrs C's blood glucose level patterns over the preceding four months. The haemoglobin A1C tests about a two to three month period, since it is based on the life of the red blood cell life span (American Diabetes Association, 1997). The chart is an additional source of information, and is part of the assessment of the patient over time.

Daily blood glucose levels are lacking secondary to Mrs C's, her husband's and her daughter's unwillingness to test Mrs C with a home glucose monitor for fear of hurting her. Mrs C is familiar with the visiting nurse services and has stated that she would welcome a visiting nurse into the home to check on her condition and her glucose level. The APN has identified barriers to home blood glucose monitoring, and is looking for ways to get more frequent measurements during this critical period.

The working diagnosis for Mrs C's muscle cramps is hypoglycaemic episodes, with hypomagnesaemia as a contributing factor. The APN's management plan is to discontinue the diuretic since it may be causing some volume depletion and electrolyte imbalances, increase high magnesium foods, and recheck the magnesium level in several weeks. If Mrs C's blood pressure rises, her ACE inhibitor anti-hypertensive medication can be increased. The reason for her hypoglycaemia appears to be secondary to one of her diabetes medications, the sulfonylurea glyburide. The APN knows that the oral sulfonylurea is long lasting, and that an elderly diabetic with hypoglycaemia who is taking a sulfonylurea may remain hypoglycaemic for several days, and can become more hypoglycaemic even without additional medication (Bloom & Shlom, 1993). Although she knows that metformin does not cause hypoglycaemia by itself, she knows that its effect is additive to the activity of the sulfonylurea (DeFronzo *et al.*, 1995).

The triage nurse tells the APN that Mrs C's blood glucose has risen to 94, and Mrs C is asking to go home to eat lunch. Both the patient and her daughter are getting restless, stating that they are not sure what all the fuss is about, since Mrs C feels fine. The APN visits Mrs C, telling her that she will be able to leave shortly, but careful plans need to be developed for the weekend to avoid further hypoglycaemia and its possibly disastrous sequelae. The APN also discusses the possibility that low blood glucose levels may be the cause of Mrs C's finger cramping. She leaves Mrs C and consults with the physician who will be covering patients over the weekend, and they decide to discontinue all diabetic medications over the weekend, encourage Mrs C to eat regularly, review the signs and symptoms of hypoglycaemia, and impress on Mrs C and her daughter the reasons that low blood glucose needs to be remedied as soon as possible if it occurs. Mrs C and her daughter are instructed to call the clinic if any symptoms of hypoglycaemia occur. A visiting nurse will check on Mrs C daily for signs and symptoms of hypoglycaemia, monitor blood glucose and blood pressure twice daily, and report daily to the provider on call. The visiting nurse will begin teaching the patient how to self monitor her blood glucose. If blood glucose levels continue to rise, the future plan is to reinstate the metformin.

In this visit with Mrs C, the APN has used advanced assessment and management skills to prioritize and attend to the needs of the patient. She has taken care of this hypoglycaemic episode, and has developed a plan for management of Mrs C's diabetes which involves the patient as well as other health care professionals. She has also continued to proceed in the search for the cause of Mrs C's finger cramping which has not yet been determined, but will continue to be evaluated over time.

Case study – insulin dependent diabetes mellitus

Ms Y, a 28 year old woman, comes to the primary care clinic for an 'urgent visit' appointment, having received no previous care at that centre. Her complaint on this visit is one of back pain and bilateral foot pain. The back pain started four days ago after she tripped getting out of an elevator and caught herself on the door frame to prevent a fall. The pain is in the thoracic area, and is dull, aching and radiates down to the sacral area. Acetaminophen helps 'a little'.

Her foot pain has had a more gradual onset over the past month. It is tingling/burning with occasional sharp, stabbing pain, worse at night. It is unaffected by the acetaminophen. Focusing on the chief complaint, the nurse practitioner attempts to get a clear description of both back and feet symptoms. She reviews the seven attributes of a symptom with Ms Y (Table 6.11).

Table 6.11 Seven attributes of pain (Bates, 1995).

---

(1) Location, does it change? Radiate?
(2) Quality of the pain/discomfort. (You may need to supply a list of descriptive nouns to assist the patient.)
(3) Its quantity or severity. Can the pain be rated on a scale? (1–10)
(4) Onset of the symptoms. When did it start? How long does it last? How often does it come?
(5) The setting in which it occurs, including environmental factors, personal activities, emotional reactions, or other contributory circumstances.
(6) Factors that make it better or worse (alleviators and aggravators).
(7) Associated manifestations.

After reviewing her symptoms, the APN goes on to review Ms Y's history. In this urgent visit setting, she knows she must quickly focus in on the medical/surgical history which may contribute to today's problem. Ms Y is comfortable enough, and answers the questions easily and with seemingly accurate recall. When the APN learns that Ms Y is a diabetic, she explores the diet and exercise history. This is an area she may have otherwise omitted in an urgent visit. However it is highly relevant here (see Table 6.12).

Table 6.12 Initial assessment.

Medical history	She has insulin dependent diabetes mellitus which was diagnosed at age 8. She was hospitalized three times for diabetic keto-acidosis. Except for one childbirth, she has had no other hospitalizations. She denies other chronic illnesses.
Medications	NPH insulin 25 u q a Acetaminophen 2 tabs q 4 hours for back pain
Diet	High in carbohydrates and fats due to food in shelter and lack of money
Exercise	Walks every day with daughter for at least 30 minutes
Social	Smokes $\frac{1}{2}$ pack per day Denies current alcohol/drug use, never used intravenous drugs Previous history of cocaine use per nostril and smoking, stopped 6 mths ago Parents live out of country, grandmother lives locally Separated from father of 2 year old daughter, due to his physical abuse of patient Lives in women's shelter for past month

In a review of systems with the diabetic patient, especially in an urgent visit situation, it is important that the APN focuses on certain areas. Although the chief complaint is back pain, it is important to quickly go over the pertinent systems with the patient with an understanding of the potential sequelae of her disease.

Late complications of diabetes develop 15–20 years after the initial onset of the disease. They include circular abnormalities affecting large and small vessels. Retinopathy is a leading cause of blindness in people less than 60 years old. Early manifestations are micro aneurysms, haemorrhages and hard exudates (rarely impair vision). Later stages include macular oedema, cotton wool spots and proliferative retinopathy (new vessels growing into the vitreous humour) causing a risk of bleeding into the vitreous humour or retinal detachment and subsequent loss of vision (Barker *et al.*, 1995).

Nephropathy is usually a later manifestation than retinopathy that may progress to persistent gross proteinuria, azotaemia, and end-stage renal disease. All of the above manifestations may be asymptomatic. Good blood pressure control may prevent or delay nephropathy.

Large vessel atherosclerosis as a complication leads to decreased circulation affecting the lower extremities. Consequently, lesions on the foot are less likely to heal. Increased infections in the feet can lead to amputation. In coronary artery disease, hyperglycaemia *may* be less of a risk factor than smoking; other risks include high lipids, hypertension and family history of coronary artery disease. Chest pain may be silent or atypical in the diabetic patient (Barker *et al.*, 1995).

The most common form of neuropathy is peripheral symmetrical poly-neuropathy which develops gradually, and is difficult if not impossible to reverse. Signs and symptoms include: numbness, tingling, dysaesthesia, 'pins and needles' which start on toes and progress up the extremity. Autonomic neuropathy affects a number of systems including genital-urinary: residual urine; vascular: orthostatic hypotension; gastro-intestinal: constipation, diarrhoea; gastroparesis: nausea/vomiting/bloating, early satiety. The APN reviews the systems with Ms Y (Table 6.13).

Table 6.13 Review of systems.

General/constitutional	She has experienced an undetermined weight loss, + fatigue, + polyuria, denies polydipsia or polyphagia
Head, eyes, ears, nose and throat	No headache, occasional blurred vision, no specks or floaters, + bleeding gums .
Cardiac/pulmonary	No chest pain, no palpitations, denies sob, + early am cough, with clear phlegm, no known TB exposure
Gastro-intestinal	She complains of a bloating sensation post-prandial, occasional constipation
Genital-urinary	Denies dysuria (+ polyuria)
Gynaecologic	Denies abnormal vaginal discharge, last menstrual period 3 months ago. Sexually inactive for 6 months
Musculoskeltal	Low back pain as described
Neurologic	Denies dizziness, one episode of tripping due to either loss of balance or obstruction of doorway. Burning sensation of feet as described. Occasional muscle weakness in legs. No loss of consciousness or seizures
Skin	Generalized dry skin, mild pruritis, no rashes

The last system to be evaluated in this patient is psychiatric, or mental status. The APN is already concerned because the patient volunteered early in the visit that she was living in a women's shelter because her boyfriend had hit her. Screening for both domestic violence and depression should be included in an encounter with every new patient. Screening for domestic violence/abuse is necessary because victims will often not reveal their situation and also may attempt to minimize or hide it. Women who may be at higher risk for domestic violence are women who are pregnant and women who have partners who have substance abuse problems. Common physical symptomatologies presented to a health care provider can be headache, abdominal pain, muscle/joint pain, fatigue, vaginal/pelvic pain and anxiety/depression. A screening mnemonic which may be used to detect violence or abuse is SAFETI (Table 6.14). Treatment issues are given in Table 6.15 (Flitcraft & Parenteau, 1995).

Table 6.14 SAFETI form (Flitcraft & Parenteau, 1995).

S: Has your partner slapped, struck or punched you?
A: Are you afraid of your partner?
F: Has your partner ever forced you to have sex?
E: Have you been emotionally or verbally abused by your partner?
T: Have you been afraid to tell someone the truth about an injury inflicted by your partner?
I: Have you been injured by your partner?

Table 6.15 Some treatment issues in a patient who is a survivor of domestic violence (Flitcraft & Parenteau, 1995).

(1) Identify the safety of the patient now
(2) Is there a child involved? Is s/he safe with either partner? Identify resources currently available
(3) Identify a willingness to seek help in leaving relationship
(4) Document any injury

Ms Y has clearly taken herself out of a dangerous situation and says she currently feels safe. She understands where to get help if she needs it and will not hesitate to call the police if threatened again. Her boyfriend does not know where she is living now. She is not concerned about the physical safety of her child, although she is concerned about the child's emotional stability.

The APN takes the opportunity to continue her evaluation of Ms Y by asking questions about depression and suicide potential. In this brief encounter the APN knows she is pressed for time but also realizes Ms Y may be at high risk. About 30% of patients seen in a general practice setting suffer from a disturbance of mood characterized by depression which may be with or without manic episodes (Barker *et al.*, 1995). Those patients who may be at high risk for depression are those who have drug or alcohol abuse problems, chronic illness, family history of depression, post-partum state, or are recovering from major surgery or a cerebral vascular accident.

The APN screens Ms Y and notes that she fits the criteria for a major depression (Table 6.16). She then evaluates her for suicide potential by saying, 'It sounds like you have been through a lot. Have you ever felt like

Table 6.16   Signs and symptoms of a major depressive episode (APA, 1994).

(1)   Depressed mood
(2)   Loss of interest or pleasure (anhedonia)
(3)   Weight loss or gain
(4)   Insomnia or hypersomnia
(5)   Psychomotor agitation retardation
(6)   Fatigue or low energy
(7)   Feelings of worthlessness or excessive guilt
(8)   Diminished ability to think or concentrate
(9)   Recurrent thoughts of death, suicidal ideation or suicide attempt

Patients must have five or more of the above during a 2 week period and one symptom must include either no. 1 or no. 2.

life is not worth living? Or that you may wish to end your life?' Ms Y promptly replies that despite all she has been through, her faith in God and love of her child give her strength to 'carry on'.

The APN compliments Ms Y on her strength and assures her that now she will move on to the physical examination and try to help her with her back pain. Although Ms Y has presented the APN with some disturbing medical and social issues, the nurse practitioner is aware that the patient's clearly stated agenda is to address her back pain. By acknowledging and addressing her patient's current concern, APN hopes to develop an ongoing relationship which may improve Ms Y's chronic illness.

She leaves the room to allow Ms Y to disrobe, which allows the APN to gather paperwork, referral slips, patient education sheets and sample medications. Table 6.17 shows details of the physical examination.

The APN's assessment and diagnoses are:

- Insulin dependent diabetes mellitus: poor control with probable peripheral neuropathy and possible diabetic amyotrophy
- Low back pain probably of musculo-skeletal origin
- History of drug abuse
- History of domestic violence and current homeless status
- Rule out major depressive episode

Since this is an 'urgent visit' the APN must prioritize her care for Ms Y. (Table 6.18 shows routine health maintenance.) She decides that the issues today are to:

- Ensure continuity of care
- Evaluate the patient's understanding of her disease and her ability to organize her life around self care (for example, how and when does she take her insulin?)

Table 6.17 Physical examination.

Ms Y is a sad-looking, thin, attractive, neatly dressed woman, who moves slowly in the examination room.

Vital signs	65 in, 118 lb, blood pressure is 120/72 mmHg, pulse is 80, temperature 98°, blood glucose 378
Head, eyes, ears, nose and throat	Pupils equal and reactive to light and accommodation, fundi show no exudates. Mouth shows well-maintained teeth with some swollen gingiva. Thyroid is smooth, non-enlarged
Cardiac	Regular heart rate and rhythm, no murmurs
Pulmonary	Lungs clear to auscultation
Abdomen	Normoactive bowel sounds, no hepatosplenomegaly, describes 'bloating' by pointing to lower epigastrium
Back	Skin clear, tender paraspinal muscles without spasm t10-L 5. No bony spinal tenderness on percussion, no costal vertebral angle tenderness
Musculoskeletal	Negative straight leg raising. Heel-toe walking performed, deep knee bend performed with difficulty. Full flexion, extension, rotation performed with some discomfort
Neurologic	Deep tendon reflexes 2+ biceps, triceps, 1+ patellar, achilles. Decreased vibratory sensation bilateral on great toe. Decreased sensation to soft and sharp touch up to malleolus bilaterally. Sensation of lower extremities intact. Some decreased sensation of anterior thigh. Muscle strength good bilaterally upper extremities, good quadriceps, hamstring strength
Peripheral vascular	Feet cool with palpable pedal pulses, some decreased hair distribution on feet/ankles
Skin	Scattered cysts on neck/jaw area. Feet: skin clear without fissures, exudates, toenails properly cut

Table 6.18 Routine health maintenance.

- Patients with dramatic chronic diseases and/or chaotic life situations often do not have routine health maintenance addressed
- Encourage smoking cessation
- Evaluate street drug abstinence
- Offer HIV testing

- Evaluate her sense of being safe
- Evaluate her suicide risk
- Treat her back pain
- Begin to evaluate her disease state
- Begin to better help her control her diabetes.

Education included in today's visit would be the availability of health care access; to review signs and symptoms of hyper- and hypoglycaemia (keeping in mind she may already have some autonomic neuropathy which could mask the signs and symptoms of hypoglycaemia); back stretching exercises and appropriate body mechanics. Collaboration plans include referrals for ophthalmology, neurology and nutrition. Also, contact with a social worker preferably today to arrange a visit to evaluate her living needs, her access to proper nutrition as well as her relationship with and the safety of her child.

Laboratory tests ordered today would include a complete blood count (an occult infection could be the cause of hyperglycaemia); haemoglobin A1C (to evaluate glucose control previous to this visit); electrolytes (to evaluate kidney function, hydration status); urine for protein, leucocyte esterase (to evaluate kidney function and possible urinary tract infection as cause of hyperglycaemia); and a pregnancy test (especially critical if planning to prescribe medications).

In considering medications for today, although a non-steroidal anti-inflammatory may be the usual drug of choice for muscle pain, you do not know her kidney function. She also has a probable peripheral neuropathy with a possible amyotrophy of the pelvic girdle. A possible alternative would be amitriptyline in addition to acetaminophen. By explaining the rationale for prescribing her the medications, the APN is also able to impress upon Ms Y her concern for the possible sequelae of her uncontrolled diabetes, which in this case may be poor kidney function. Non-medical treatment for her back pain is suggested as well. The APN gives Ms Y instructions on back stretching exercises and encourages moist heat to the area.

It is unclear why Ms Y's glucose is high, and how long it has been so. The most frequent causes of worsening hyperglycaemia are inadequate insulin dose; increased caloric intake; failure to take properly; occult infection; severe emotional stress; use of corticosteroids; coronary ischaemia; insulin resistance; and Somogyi phenomenon.

The APN believes Ms Y's hyperglycaemia is probably due to poor caloric intake, stress, and possibly an inadequate insulin dose. She discusses with Ms Y home glucose monitoring, and the logistics of performing it in the shelter. Since Ms Y has had extensive experience with a glucometer, they decide to equip her with one to take home.

The APN creates a plan with Ms Y to maintain telephone contact at a certain time of day. Ms Y provides the APN with the number of the shelter and the director's name.

It is determined that Ms Y will have morning and evening doses of insulin, increased slowly over time, based on her fasting and 4 PM glucose. Follow-up visit goals are centred around continuing efforts at glucose control, continued patient education about the sequelae of prolonged hyperglycaemia and education about proper foot care. Previous medical records would be very helpful in understanding this patient, although not critical to her care today.

Conclusion

The three cases offer slightly different scenarios of the process of health assessment in the context of management of chronic health problems. All three point out the need for an initial assessment and continuing re-assessment in the clinical encounter between a patient and an advanced practice nurse. The health issues for these patients were not clear-cut, as is frequently the case in real life. In each of the cases, the reality of the patients' lives is linked with both the causes of their health problems and the management of those problems. The elicitation of information, through interview and physical examination, is balanced by the evaluation of the data by the advanced practice nurse to offer comprehensive, holistic care.

References

American Diabetes Association (1997) Clinical Practice Recommendations 1997. *Diabetes Care*, **20** (Suppl. 1).

APA (1994) *Diagnostic and Statistical Manual of Mental Disorders*, 4th edn. American Psychiatric Association, Washington DC.

Barker, L.R., Burton, J.R. & Zieve, P.D. (1995) *Principles of Ambulatory Medicine*, 4th edn. Williams and Wilkins, Baltimore.

Bates, B. (1995) Table 11 and reference list. *A Guide to Physical Examination and History Taking* (6th edn). J.B. Lippincott, Philadelphia.

Beaser, R.S. & Hill, J.V.C. (1995) *The Joslin Guide to Diabetes: A program for managing your treatment*, pp. 170–6. Simon and Schuster, New York.

Bloom, H.G. & Shlom, E.A. (1993) *Drug Prescribing for the Elderly*, pp. 161–3. Raven Press, New York.

Brykczynski, K. (1985) Exploring the clinical practice of nurse practitioners. Doctoral dissertation, University of California, San Francisco. Dissertation Abstracts International, 46, 3789B (University Microfilms No. DA86-00592).

DeFronzo, R.A., Goodman, A.M. *et al.* (1995) Efficacy of metformin in patients with non-insulin-dependent diabetes mellitus. *New England Journal of Medicine*, **333** (9), 541–9.

Flitcraft, A. & Parenteau, K. (1995) *Project Safe: A healthcare professional's guide to domestic violence.* Domestic Violence Training Project, New Haven, CT.

Goroll, A., May, L. & Mulley, A. (1995) *Primary Care Medicine: Office Evaluation and Management of the Adult Patient.* J.B. Lippincott, Philadelphia.

JNC (1993) The Fifth Report of the Joint National Committee on Detection, Evaluation, and Treatment of High Blood Pressure. *Archives of Internal Medicine*, **153**, 154–87.

Margolis, S. & Klag, M. (1996) Hypertension. *The Johns Hopkins White Papers*. Johns Hopkins Press, Baltimore.

Rifkin, H. & Porte, D. (1990) *Diabetes Mellitus: Theory and practice.* Elsevier, New York.

Speicher, C.E. (1993) *The Right Test: A Physician's Guide to Laboratory Medicine.* W.B. Saunders, Philadelphia.

Wood, M. (1996) Current considerations in patients with coexisting diabetes and hypertension. *Nurse Practitioner*, **21** (4), 19–31.

Further reading

Alderman, M., Grim, R.Jr, Swales, J.D. & Weart, C.W. (1995) Treating hypertension: which drugs first? *Patient Care*, **29** (16), 72–6, 83, 86 passim.

Butler, M.J. (1995) Domestic violence: a nursing imperative. *Journal of Holistic Nursing*, **13** (1), 54–69.

Haire-Joshu, D. (ed.) (1992) *Management of Diabetes Mellitus: Perspectives of care across the life span.* Mosby-Year Book, Boston.

Harper, K. & Forker, A. (1992) Antihypertensive therapy: current issues and challenges. *Postgraduate Medicine*, **91** (6), 163–93.

Chapter 7

Assessing Competence

Sue Lillyman

Introduction

Competence is a concept that is widely used within all aspects of nursing, midwifery and health visiting. As the practitioner moves through their career they are deemed competent at differing levels of practice. At initial registration the practitioner is competent to practise as a qualified nurse or midwife, and following further experience and practice they move to proficient and expert practice (Benner, 1984). The United Kingdom Central Council for Nurses, Midwives and Health Visitors (UKCC, 1990) identified higher levels of practice as specialist and advanced. It is the assessment of these higher levels of practice that has proved difficult for the practitioner and the educationalist to define and measure. The concept of what constitutes competence at a higher level, and the assessment, require further exploration.

This chapter will attempt to identify what is meant by the competent specialist and advanced practitioner and offer some criteria on which this competence can be assessed.

The problem with competence

Recent pressure to define competence has come from the European Union: to relate qualifications and the individual's ability to perform tasks at a given level (Weightman, 1994). With the introduction of the *Post Registration, Education and Practice* requirements the process of continual development has become a requirement of all practitioners in order to maintain their registration. The definition of competence and therefore developing practice has proved problematic for all involved in education and practice. The increase in academic criteria and the continual demand to improve levels of practice from the organization have led to increased professional autonomy and accountability for the practitioner (Jones, 1994). In order to address these issues the profession needs to identify at what level a practitioner is performing. Once the level of practice is determined then the process of working towards a higher level of competence will lead to the identification of the specialist and advanced practitioner.

Patients expect that the most appropriate care will be delivered in the 'most skilled manner' and by the 'best able' to deliver it (Clay, 1987). In order for the practitioner to deliver the best care the nurse, midwife or health visitor has to be a competent practitioner in their area and level of care. To identify this practitioner several questions/issues need to be addressed:

(1) The notion of competence
(2) At what level is a specialist and advanced practitioner to be assessed as competent?
(3) How can the 'best able' be assessed as competent in delivering care?

The notion of competence

Coit-Butler (1978) stated that there is no universal agreement among educators as to what constitutes competence. This debate continues two decades later with no clear and agreed definition. Competence is often judged as a continuum and measured against incompetence. The concept of competence in practice is based on set standards, using an identified criterion. The practitioner is deemed as being not competent by not achieving the desired standard. This definition relies on the development of agreed set competencies that are then identified at differing levels of practice.

At the point of registration the practitioner gains their licence to practice and are qualified in a given area of competence. The level of that practice is deemed as safe practice. The English National Board for Nurses, Midwives and Health Visitors identify competence as 'the ability to perform particular activities to a prescribed standard' (ENB, 1993, section 6.4). On qualification a nurse is judged via a variety of practical and academic assessment criteria to have achieved the level of competent practice. The UKCC (1986) stated that the new registered practitioner is:

'competent to assess the need for care, provide care, monitor and evaluate and to do this in institutional and non-institutional settings.'

The individual practitioner, having undergone a process of education and assessment, is judged by the profession to have attained an agreed level of competence at which they continue to perform.

Following registration the practitioner is required to continue to demonstrate that they have developed and maintained their level of competence. As stated by the UKCC (1994):

'The continuing demands and complexity of professional practice require registered practitioners to not only maintain and develop their professional knowledge and competence, but to do so in the interests of patient and client care.'

This has now been identified in the *Post Registration, Education and Practice* requirements (UKCC, 1990) which demand that:

'all nurses, midwives and health visitors must demonstrate that they have maintained and developed their clinical competence.'

The *Code of Professional Conduct* (UKCC, 1992) backs this up with the statement that:

'all nurses, midwives and health visitors must endeavour always to achieve, maintain and develop knowledge, skill and competence.'

The code is concerned with the minimum level of performance to ensure high quality of care. Each document refers to competence primarily at the registration level (UKCC, 1986), and the post-registration level (UKCC, 1990, 1992, 1994). They do not, however, identify how following registration the practitioner develops his/her competence in practice at a higher level, and the area of assessment of the competent specialist and advanced practice is not identified in these documents.

The preregistration nurse and midwife progresses from, as Benner (1984) identifies, the 'novice' to 'competent' practitioner and is usually assessed against incompetence. So how can we define competence? There is no agreement as to exactly what may or may not be considered instances of competence. Furnham (1993) notes that the concept is both multi-dimensional and somewhat ambiguous.

Competence as behaviour

Competent practice is often identified as an observable behaviour. This behavioural approach is demonstrated in the traditional nurse education programmes (Pashley & Henry, 1990). The competencies are formulated into sets of performance criteria that can be measured by directly observing the practitioner's behaviour. Many pre-registration curriculums have based their course competencies on the behavioural competencies. In order to identify the level of practice, taxonomies such as Bloom (1956) are utilized. Individual practitioners move from the lower level of knowledge to the higher level of evaluation, from observing to performing skills. These taxonomies identify for the assessor the move from novice to competent practice. They rely on the measurement of the behavioural performance at the given level of the taxonomy. Failure to achieve these levels results in incompetence and non registration.

The behaviourist approach describes actions, behaviour or outcomes performed by the individual. The behavioural competence can be assessed using an identified guide or performance outcome chart. Lillyman (1997), however, notes that this model fails to measure the underlying cognitive and affective skills that the individual requires to practice effectively. It also fails to consider any bias of the observer. Norris (1991) argues that the concept of competence places a greater emphasis on the assessment of performance rather than knowledge. The Unit for the Development of Adult Continuing Education report (1989) agrees as they identify that the problem of competence is concerned with what people can do rather than what they know. Messick (1984) notes that competencies are also related to the individual's potential and not just demonstrated behaviour. The behavioural objectives or outcomes approach fails to address the total notion of competence in practice and therefore is not appropriate to use as a definition when referring to the specialist and advanced practitioner. Norris (1991) states that if competence is about what people can do, then at first sight it appears to circumvent the issue of what people know. It shifts that balance firmly in the direction of practice and away from theory. The notion of competence as performance follows the same arguments.

Norris (1991) goes on to suggest that when writing competencies they should be easy to understand, permit direct observation, be expressed as outcomes and be transferable from setting to setting. He suggests they be straightforward, flexible and meet national as opposed to local standards. However, Gonczi (1994) argues that attempting to make the process simple and clear fails in other respects: it ignores the underlying attributes and group processes that the individual possesses. Competencies become atheoretical and conservative and ignore the complexity of performance and the role of professional judgement in the real world.

Worth-Butler *et al.* (1994) note the confusion about competencies as they believe these involve not only behaviour which can be measured, but also attributes such as attitudes, values, judgemental abilities and personal dispositions. Their definition of competence is people who have learned an adequate set of skills and knowledge to do their job satisfactorily. A capable professional is someone who is able to draw on that repertoire of skills and knowledge in different ways and in different contexts and to perform in a way that is recognized as competent. They fail, however, to identify the levels of competence in practice. Other authors suggest that it is more complex and involves other aspects, including cognitive, experiential, personal and scientific knowledge (Johns, 1995).

As identified earlier there is considerable confusion between the terms competence and performance. Some authors suggest that to measure competence is a complex issue whereas to measure performance is easier. Sternberg (1990) notes that since competence is not an objective phenomenon concerned with perceived skills, it cannot be measured, but he argues that performance is open to measurement. The English National Board for Nurses, Midwives and Health Visitors regulations for courses approval (ENB, 1993) reflect this, with reference only to competence that is 'the ability to perform particular activities to prescribed standards'. Thompson *et al.* (1990) question the expertise of these individuals as the actual performance, ability to perform, or simply a domain knowledge.

While (1994) notes the confusion between the field of competence and performance and suggests that there should be a greater emphasis placed in the real life clinical setting rather than on behavioural competence measured at one performance. Henderson (1992) states that central to the whole process is the need to be a safe practitioner.

Competence as critical thinking

Another aspect of competence has been introduced into the competency debate. Howstein *et al.* (1996) state that the ability to think critically in increasingly hypothesized situations plays an important role in a nurse's ability to function competently in a complex health care setting. Bauens and Gerharch (1987) and Harbison (1991) argue that the ability to think critically and analytically underlies much of competent nursing practice. Watson and Glaser (1980) state that critical thinking is a composite of attitudes, knowledge and skills, while Facione *et al.* (1994) suggest that both the use of cognitive skills and the dispositions to think critically can enhance the clinical judgement process. Knowledge, according to Conger and Mezza (1996), goes beyond the acquisition of facts and rules to an active process of deliberation, interpretation and reflection until cognitive structures are formed. These arguments may lead us closer to identifying and assessing competent specialist and advanced practitioners at differing levels of practice. If critical thinking can be analysed and assessed, the move towards identifying the competent practitioner may be possible.

In Australia the nursing field is working towards an 'integrated' or 'holistic' approach to competence (Gonczi, 1994). Competence is perceived as a complex structuring of attributes needed for intelligent performance. In specific situations, incorporating professional judgement, reflective practice, ethics and values may also suggest there is more than one way of practising competently. Cash (1995) notes that Benner (1984) bases her position on the difference between practical and theoretical knowledge – 'knowing how' and 'knowing that' – the difference between prepositional knowledge, knowing that, and the ability to perform, knowing how. Benner's argument is related to intuition and also has its place in critical thinking.

Types of tests discussed by Howstein *et al.* (1996) to measure critical thinking include the Watson–Glaser clinical thinking appraisal, California critical thinking skills test, Ennis–Weir critical thinking essay test, and Cornell critical thinking test. These provide a measurement tool.

Levels of competence

At what level is a specialist and advanced practitioner to be assessed as competent? While (1994) notes that there is an increasing body of empirical literature which indicates that apparently competent registered practitioners frequently do not always perform at an adequate level.

The qualities, skills and knowledge of a 'good' nurse have altered over the past few decades (Jones, 1994). Practitioners have had to adapt and develop with a changing health service. Differing levels of practice have emerged. Patterson and Haddad (1992) and Benner (1984) state that nurses practise at different levels of expertise regardless of their specialist area or level of care setting. According to While (1994) there is a difference between what an individual should be able to do at an expected level of achievement and what they actually do in the real life setting. Schon (1987) and Benner (1984) identify that it is the artistry of the practice that differentiates between the levels of a competent and expert practitioner.

For the specialist and advanced practitioner the journey through levels of practice is not so well defined. This leads to problems of assessment, as already discussed. The entrance for these expert practitioners starts from what Benner would refer to as an 'expert' practitioner position. Expert, however, is often related to time spent in practice, but Jarvis (1994) notes that time in practice does not automatically gain knowledge. Practitioners may rely on outdated or inappropriate practices.

The UKCC in their *Post Registration Education and Practice* document (UKCC, 1990) refer to the specialist and advanced practitioner as a practitioner who has an obligation to achieve a higher level of competence in practice, developing and maintaining their practice.

With the introduction of higher levels of practice, nursing and midwifery education responded with the pre-registration curriculum. To replace the 'one off' assessment of performance, the continual practical assessment was introduced. This allowed the student to demonstrate a continual level of performance over a period and in a variety of clinical environments. However, this assessment is often based on the observation of the behavioural outcome that is measured.

Sutton and Smith (1995) note that consistency in enacting a range of specific skills and functioning within similar nursing situations enhances a practitioner's opportunity to develop expertise. Benner (1984) identifies clinical expertise exhibited by experts as an in-depth knowledge of clinical practice. Benner fails to identify how individuals change and move from one level of expertise to another. Girot (1995) notes that it is critical thinking by the qualified practitioner that values the level of work that is being performed. Measuring critical thinking recognizes and justifies what they have to offer, as distinct from their non-professional assistants. Greenwood and King (1995) in their study identified that 'expert' and 'novice' orthopaedic nurses actually used the same level of concepts and critical reasoning. Both groups were physically orientated and the reasoning of both was consistent with the medical model. Benner (1984) disagrees with this in her notion of the expert practitioner level differing from the novice practitioner.

Norris (1991), when talking about standards, refers back to the performance issues and states that they are thought about as levels of achievement or performance. There is required the designation and justification of a criterion level below which performance is deemed unsatisfactory and above which mastery is attained. The level of standard designed is a desirable or necessary level of attainment. Glass (1978) stated that the idea of standards in educational assessment is connected with criterion referenced testing. Norris (1991) notes that knowledge evidenced in action appeals to those who want to maintain the primacy of performance evidence in the assessment of competence. He suggests that competence should be seen as professional judgement resting as much on tacit understanding as it does on prepositional knowledge. The complexity is identified when the range of activities a person performs appropriately and effectively is deemed to be competent. At what level is the performance assessed for the specialist and advanced practitioner? Lillyman (1997) identifies the added problem of consistency of maintaining and developing that competent practice. She argues that the one off measurement on a given programme will not ensure continued development over time. Deeming an individual competent may lead to poor practice if the individual does not continue to develop or maintain that practice.

Any criteria used to assess competence must reduce subjectivity, provide consistency and identify the level of practice. Assessment of competence may be identified as a judgement by another. Competence in clinical practice, as well as being assessed, must also be transferable to differing areas of practice and achievable by the individual practitioner. If nurses, midwives, health visitors and educationalists are concerned with competence, the assessment of clinical competence continues to be a concern for all whatever the level of care the practitioner provides.

Chickadonz and Perry (1985) suggest that the specialist nurse fails to explicate the specialist nursing knowledge associated with each field of practice. They suggest that he or she has only taken aspects of knowledge and skills which were previously the province of doctors and much debate surrounds this issue. The definition and understanding as to what constitutes the practice of the specialist and advanced practitioner is relevant in the provision of assessment tools that are used to measure that practice. Watson (1991) notes the difficulty in measuring experience. Qualitative standards or criteria judgements are based on subjective professional judgements based on experience.

To overcome some of these arguments there has been a move to introduce the objective structures clinical evaluation as identified by Bujack *et al.* (1991). This system is derived from the medical approach to assessment, in a safe environment out of the clinical setting where the practitioner encounters simulated examples of nursing practice. This method attempts to measure the practitioner's knowledge and skills and their use in planning, implementing and evaluating care in a single patient encounter. This, however, was questioned by Ross *et al.* (1988) as they felt it did not reflect the clinical reality of nursing. It also fails to measure the consistency of that practice.

The specialist practitioner is defined by the UKCC (1994) as 'a practitioner who exercises higher levels of judgement and discretion in clinical care'. The method of accrediting these individuals to become specialist practitioners relies presently on the academic standing of the individual and the consistency and performance of their practice, the specialist practitioner having gained degree level education and advanced practitioners master's and higher qualifications.

The clinical nurse specialist, according to Miller (1995), has an increasing level of knowledge which may cover a broad field. Their role, according to Miller, is:

- Clinical expert
- Resources/consultant
- Educator
- Change agent
- Researcher
- Advocate

Each role will require some level of assessment of their competence to perform these roles in the clinical field. It would not fulfil all the requirements if the academic level were taken without identifying the level of practice. Benner (1984) describes ways in which an expert can be identified as based on those who possess intuition and time spent in practice. She describes a competent nurse as one who has been in post for 2–3 years, and more time in practice for the expert. She notes that the more expert the practitioner becomes, the more he or she breaks the scene down into important elements and imparts a sense of fluidity and relevance in the use of the language. Benner argues that this level of analysis enabled her to describe the performance characteristics at each level of development.

Growth and expertise are developmental; the expert practitioner is strongly intuitive and expert practice is by the approval of a specific group that is empowered to give it. The concept of expert remains arbitrary and can prove inconsistent. Cash (1995) notes that Benner's model retreats into the validation of practice by authority and tradition.

Sutton and Smith (1995) postulate that advanced practice differs from expert and specialist nursing practice and that this is evident in the different ways in which advanced nurse practitioners think, see and experience nursing practice.

Competence and education

Girot's (1995) growing concern in nursing in recent years is the ability of practitioners to keep pace with changing developments in health care. Educational literature frequently refers to competence as the outcome of educational programmes. While (1994) notes that nurse education continues to assume that competence is an adequate criterion of proficiency for professional registration, with no acknowledgement of the potential difference between competence and future performance in the real life setting. The International Council of Nursing in 1992 stated that 'all nurses require ongoing continuing education to maintain their professional competency in the rapidly changing health field'. Yoder-Wise (1996) argues that time spent does not equal knowledge gained or ensure competent performance. Patterson and Haddad (1992) argue that the level at which practitioners perform is not reliant on individual education.

Continuing education requirements, with few exceptions, ask only that licences show the practitioners have attended approved continuing educational courses (Pew, 1995). Benner's (1984) model of skill acquisition is used as a framework underpinning the Project 2000 curriculum (UKCC, 1987) and is a recommended structure for post-registration education and practice (UKCC, 1990). Elio and Scharf (1990) suggested that a number of studies and models of novice-to-expert differences have intimated that the expert not only knows more than the novice but there are qualitative difference in how experts and novices organize their knowledge and use it during problem solving.

Experience measured in quantitative terms is widespread but in qualitative terms is less well understood; however, the latter may prove more important (Watson, 1991). Fergusson (1984) suggests that Project 2000 may not be developing expertise in the student due to the separation of the practice of nursing from its discipline and the reliance on academic disciplines for scientific knowledge. Noyes (1995) notes that Benner's model of skills acquisition appears flawed as the model promotes recognition of problems, rather than identification and a problem solving process, endangering explicit clinical expertise. Howstein *et al.* (1996) found in their study that the level of education was positively related to critical thinking. The other argument, according to Watson (1991), is that knowledge is familiarity gained by experience.

Assessing competence

The final question is how to assess the competent practitioner. Assessment of competence needs addressing in relation to all levels of nursing, midwifery and health visiting practice from the novice to the advanced practitioner. Gonczi (1994) argues that assessors make judgements based on evidence gathered from the performance(s). It is about whether an individual meets criteria specific in a profession's competency standard. Competence, when reviewing all the arguments discussed, remains complex; it cannot be observed directly, it can only be inferred from performance. Greater emphasis is required on the application and synthesis of knowledge in an attempt to assess the role of other attributes in professional performance.

Benner (1984) states that 'measurement can be only as productive and accurate as the competencies selected to be measured'. Mozingo *et al.* (1995) notes that competence levels may be affected by self esteem, anxiety and stress, academic experiences, demographic characteristics and availability of good role models. Assessment is not just attaining a competent level but raises the issue of how to demonstrate the ability to prove consistently competence at a given level (Lillyman, 1997). While (1994) also notes serious shortcomings in much competence assessment; he argues it is dependent on inferences derived from limited observation.

The profession therefore needs to identify who will do the assessing. As nursing moves forward, the forerunners of the specialist and advanced practitioners are entering into higher levels of practice and academic study. The educationalist measures the academic levels, but who will measure the competent practitioner? If these individuals are the first in practice the profession will need to identify their assessors in practice. The most likely candidates for this assessment are our medical colleagues. This, however, leads to problems of its own as specialist and advanced practice attempts to move away from the medical model. With the introduction of the policy for reducing junior doctors' hours, there is a danger that practitioners will move towards a mini doctors role and competence based on medical performances. The profession needs to address the use of medical colleagues in assessing further development and provide appropriate training for those already deemed experts in their field of care to develop skills in assessing and educating others. Gonczi (1994) notes the value of competence-based practice. It enables us to come closer to assessing what we want to assess – the capacity of the professional to integrate knowledge, values, attitudes and skills in the world of practice – and this must not be lost through inappropriate assessors.

Conclusion

One of the main arguments throughout this chapter has been the definition of competence. In order to identify and assess the specialist and advanced practitioner as being competent in practice, to develop appropriate tools and judge their level of practice, the definition of a competent practitioner will need to be sought. Do professionals want to continue down the academic line of deeming competence of the specialist and advanced practitioner via higher qualifications? Is the behaviourist model of observing performance, or the assessment of the critical thinking ability of the individual practitioner, appropriate for the specialist and advanced practitioner?

It may be argued that there is a need at the specialist and advanced practitioner level to utilize a combination of these approaches in identifying competence in practice. The practitioner should be required to demonstrate performance with underpinning knowledge that individuals can reflect on. The practitioner should identify through critical thinking their underpinning scientific and experiential knowledge at an identified level in practice.

References

Bauens, E. & Gerharch, G. (1987) The use of the Watson-Glaser critical thinking appraisal to predict success in baccalaureate nursing program. *Journal of Nursing Education*, **26** (7), 278–81.

Benner, P. (1984) *From Novice to Expert: Excellence and Power in Clinical Nursing Practice*. Addison Wesley, Menlo Park, California.

Bloom, B. (1956) *Taxonomy of Educational Objectives*. David Mackay, New York.

Bujack, L., McMillian, M., Dwyer, J. & Hazelton, M. (1991) Assessing comprehensive nursing performance: the objective structured clinical assessment (OSCA) Part 1. Development of the assessment strategy. *Nurse Education Today*, **11**, 179–84.

Cash, K. (1995) Benner and expertise in nursing: a critique. *International Journal of Nursing Studies*, **32** (6), 527–34.

Chickadonz, G.H. & Perry, A.M. (1985) Clinical generalisation: perspectives for the future. In: *Current Issues in Nursing*, 2nd edn (eds H. Grace & J. McCloskey). Blackwell Science, Oxford.

Clay, T. (1987) *Nurses Power and Politics*. Heinemann, London.

Coit-Butler, F. (1978) The concept of competence: an operational definition. *Educational Technology*, **18**, 7–16.

Conger, M. & Mezza, I. (1996) Fostering critical thinking in nursing students in the clinical setting. *Nurse Educator,* **21** (3), 11–15.

Elio, R. & Scharf, P. (1990) Modelling novice to expert shifts in problem solving strategy and knowledge organisation. *Cognitive Science,* **14**, 579–639.

ENB (1993) *Regulations and Guidelines for the Approval of Institutions and Courses.* English National Board for Nursing, Midwifery and Health Visiting, London.

Facione, N., Facione, P. & Sanchez, C. (1994) Critical thinking disposition as a measure of competent clinical judgement: the development of the Californian critical thinking disposition inventory. *Journal of Nursing Education,* **33** (8), 345–50.

Fergusson, M. (1984) Undergraduating nursing curriculum building: an exploration into the 'science' requirement. *Journal of Advanced Nursing,* **9**, 197–204.

Furnham, A. (1993) Competence to practice medicine. In: *Professional Competence and Quality Assurance in the Caring Professions* (ed. R. Ellis). Chapman and Hall, London.

Girot, E. (1995) Preparing practitioners for advanced academic study: the development of critical thinking. *Journal of Advanced Nursing,* **21**, 387–94.

Glass, G.V. (1978) Standards and criteria. *Journal of Education Measurement,* **15**, 237–61.

Gonczi, A. (1994) Competency based assessment in the professions in Australia. *Assessment in Education,* **1**, 27–44.

Greenwood, J. & King, M. (1995) Some surprising similarities in the clinical reasoning of 'expert' and 'novice' orthopaedic nurses. *Journal of Advanced Nursing,* **22**, 907–91.

Harbison, J. (1991) Clinical decision making in nursing. *Journal of Advanced Nursing,* **16**, 404–7.

Henderson, C. (1992) Safe, competent practitioners: developing a scheme of continuous practical assessments. *Modern Midwife,* **2** (6), 8–10.

Howstein, M., Bilodeau, K. & Good, G. (1996) Factors associated with critical thinking among nurses. *Journal of Continuing Education in Nursing,* **27** (3), 100–103.

Jarvis, P. (1994) Learning practical knowledge. *Journal of Further and Higher Education,* **12**, 3–10.

Johns, C. (1995) The value of reflective practice for nursing. *Journal of Clinical Studies,* **4**, 23–30.

Jones, L. (1994) *The Social Context of Health and Health Work.* Macmillan, London.

Lillyman, S. (1997) Credentialling in health care. In: *Excellence in Health Care Management* (eds A. Morton Cooper & M. Bamford). Blackwell, London.

Messick, S. (1984) The psychology of educational measurement. *Journal of Educational Measurement,* **21**, 215–38.

Miller, S. (1995) The clinical nurse specialist: a way forward. *Journal of Advanced Nursing* **22**, 494–501.

Mozingo, J., Thomas, S. & Brooks, E. (1995) Factors associated with perceived competency levels of graduating seniors in baccalaureate nursing programmes. *Journal of Nursing Education,* **34** (3), 115–22.

Norris, N. (1991) The trouble with competence. *Journal of Education,* **21** (3), 331–41.

Noyes, J. (1995) An explanation of the differences between expert and novice performance in the administration of an intramuscular injection of an analgesic agent to a patient in pain. *Journal of Advanced Nursing,* **22**, 800–807.

Pashley, G. & Henry, C. (1990) Carving out the nineties. *Nursing Times*, **86** (3), 45–6.

Patterson, C. & Haddad, B. (1992) The advanced nurse practitioner: common attributes. *Canadian Journal of Nursing Administration*, **5** (4), 18–22.

Pew (1995) *Reforming Health Care Workforce Regulation: Policy Consideration for the 21st Century*. Pew Health Professions Commission, San Francisco.

Ross, M., Carroll, G., Knight, J., Chamberlain, M., Fothergill-Bourbonnais, F. & Linton, J. (1988) Using the OSCE to measure clinical skills performance in nursing. *Journal of Advanced Nursing*, **13**, 45–56.

Schon, D. (1987) *Educating the Reflective Practitioner*. Jossey Bass, San Francisco.

Sternberg, R. (1990) Prototypes of competence in incompetence. In: *Competence Considered* (eds R. Sternberg & J. Kalligan), pp. 117–45. Yale University Press, Connecticut.

Sutton, F. & Smith, C. (1995) Advanced nursing practice: new ideas and new perspectives. *Journal of Advanced Nursing*, **21**, 1037–43.

Thompson, G., Ryan, S.A. & Kitzman, H. (1990) Expertise the basis for expert system development. *Advances in Nursing Science*, **13** (2), 1–10.

UDACE (1989) *Understanding Competence: a Development Paper*. The Unit for the Development of Adult Continuing Education, Northants.

UKCC (1986) *Project 2000: A New Preparation for Practice*. United Kingdom Central Council for Nurses, Midwives and Health Visitors, London.

UKCC (1987) *The Final Proposals, Project Paper 9*. United Kingdom Central Council for Nurses, Midwives and Health Visitors, London.

UKCC (1990) *The Report of Post Registration Education and Practice Project*. United Kingdom Central Council for Nurses, Midwives and Health Visitors, London.

UKCC (1992) *Professional Code of Conduct*. United Kingdom Central Council for Nurses, Midwives and Health Visitors, London.

UKCC (1994) *Standards of Education and Practice Following Registration*. United Kingdom Central Council for Nurses, Midwives and Health Visitors, London.

Watson, S. (1991) An analysis of the concept of experience. *Journal of Advanced Nursing*, **16**, 1117–21.

Watson, G. & Glaser, E. (1980) Watson Glaser Critical Thinking Appraisal Manual, Cleveland. Cited in *Critical thinking as an educational outcome* (1996) (J. Whitlow, L. Strer & K. Johnson). *Nurse Education*, **21** (3), 25–31.

Weightman, J. (1994) *Competencies in Action*. Institute of Personnel and Development, London.

While, A. (1994) Competence versus performance: which is more important? *Journal of Advanced Nursing*, **20**, 525–31.

Worth-Butler, M., Murphy, R. & Fraser, D. (1994) Towards an integrated model of competence. *Midwifery*, **10**, 225–31.

Yoder-Wise, P. (1996) Continuing education: continuing competence. *Editorial Journal of Continuing Education in Nursing*, **27** (3), 99.

Part 2
Specialist Practice

Chapter 8
Specialist Practice in the UK

Paula McGee

Introduction

Specialist practice calls on the practitioner to 'exercise higher levels of judgement and discretion in clinical care' (UKCC, 1994). Such nurses are expected to undertake more complex decision-making than professional practitioners and to 'improve standards of care through supervision of practice, clinical nursing audit, developing and leading practice, contributing to research, teaching and supporting professional colleagues' (UKCC, 1994). In order to achieve this level of practice the individual must concentrate on a particular field and undergo appropriate education which will in future be at degree level.

This British view of specialist practice is very similar to that adopted by the American Nurses Association (Girard, 1987). In both countries notions about specialist practice are based on the following needs:

- To utilize the expertise of experienced nurses, recognizing their individual contributions to patient care. All nurses are not the same and specialist practice provides opportunities for those with particular abilities or interests. Through this, new fields of practice are opened up, for example HIV/AIDS nursing, and new professional knowledge is generated.
- To value clinical practice. This is the proper work of nurses (The Nuffield Provincial Hospitals Trust, 1954) and without it nursing has no focus and no purpose. Valuing clinical practice provides career opportunities which maintain contact with patients. Thus the experienced nurse should no longer be faced with a choice between going into management or becoming a tutor. Specialist practice should provide the option of deepening knowledge and skill in direct relation to patient care.
- To recognize that initial professional education is not enough for the complexity of modern nursing. Meeting the needs of patients requires some nurses to adopt multifaceted roles which require further professional education and training.

● To differentiate between working in a specialty and being a specialist. Working in a specialty is part of professional practice and may be a stepping stone to career development. For example, an individual may take a staff nurse post in a specialty to determine whether he or she likes this particular field of practice or simply to gain some experience in that type of nursing. However, working in that field, even for 20 years, does not make the nurse a specialist. In 20 years the nurse may have provided care for very similar patients and be adept in meeting their needs but he or she will still lack breadth of experience, depth of knowledge and the skills required to lead or develop practice, all of which are the hallmark of a specialist practitioner.

Working in a specialty is a stage in becoming a specialist practitioner in that it enables the nurse to gain some experience and maybe even undertake a specialized course. In order to progress, the nurse needs a broad range of experience, in a variety of settings, which facilitates the development of advanced, transferable skills specific to the client group concerned. Beyond this there is no set pathway. Each specialist practitioner is, at the moment, free to develop his or her own pathway but will have to satisfy the UKCC that it has enabled the individual to meet the requirements of specialist practice.

A survey by McGee *et al.* (1996) showed that most specialist practitioners do in fact conform to the dimensions of the role set out by the UKCC and in North American literature. However, each role is to some extent unique depending on the field of practice and the individual postholder. The following five chapters, in Part 2 of this book, examine five examples of specialist practice roles: HIV/AIDS nursing, matron of an independent hospital, cultural liaison officer, nutrition nurse specialist and lecturer practitioner. These are compared and contrasted in relation to the sub-roles of researcher, educator, care giver, consultant, leader and manager. It must be emphasized that each specialist presents only some aspects of his/her role rather than a comprehensive account of their work.

Care giver

The specialist nurse must be an expert practitioner, one who 'knows what needs to be achieved, based on mature and situational discrimination, but also knows how to achieve the goal' (Dreyfus & Dreyfus, 1996). It is this discriminatory ability which distinguishes the expert from other practitioners, because he or she is able to identify differences in situations which appear to be similar. To arrive at this stage the nurse must pass through several stages of development in which he or she depends on rules, but on becoming expert the practitioner is able to move away from rules towards a more intuitive approach (Benner, 1984). The ability to provide expert care is essential if the specialist practitioner is to be taken seriously by other members of staff, but the activities actually performed by the specialist will vary depending on the skills of the professional practitioners involved.

In this context Helen Arrowsmith, as a nutrition nurse specialist (Chapter 12), undertakes the insertion of certain types of line for patient feeding. She does so, not just because she has the skills, but because, as an expert practitioner, she is less likely to introduce infection. She is also able to apply other knowledge and skills in caring for the patient. Once the line is in place, it is cared for either by the patient, the family or nurses, all of whom have been taught by Helen Arrowsmith. In contrast Elizabeth Alsbury is a surgical nursing specialist (Chapter 13). She is involved in direct care through her work in the pre-admission clinic where she has been able to spearhead a new development in practice. Her role contributed directly to the success of the venture even though in time, when it is running smoothly, other staff may take over certain aspects of the work. In her role as a ward sister she is also involved in direct care which enables her to remain in touch with the needs of both patients and staff, who can approach her informally.

Both these practitioners are easily accessible to the patients and staff with whom they work. Their physical presence in the workplace means that they can act as role models, demonstrate or explain things, identify patient and staff needs and support individuals in crisis (Menard, 1987; Koetters, 1989; Heffline, 1992). Thus the specialist practitioner's involvement in direct care differs from that of the professional practitioner who performs the ongoing nursing activities. Specialist care is linked to specific types of intervention for particular clients, groups of patients and staff and depends on the needs of the organization. In setting up such posts, therefore, managers and staff would be well advised to consider what it is they believe a specialist can contribute to direct care, what expertise they already have as professional practitioners and how this could be enhanced by a specialist. However, it is clear from this discussion that the specialist nurse must have firm links with practice as a basis for the other aspects of the role.

Teacher

As an expert practitioner with in-depth knowledge of the practice area, the specialist nurse is involved in teaching others. This requires the nurse to have a sound knowledge of the principles of teaching and learning, and skills needed to apply this in meeting the educational needs of diverse professional groups such as nurses, medical staff and dietitians as well as patients and their carers (Meyer, 1987). All the specialist nurses in Part 2 have a specific teaching qualification such as the Certificate of Education or the ENB course 998, in order to develop their teaching role.

Specialists can use different strategies for promoting learning. For example, in her clinical work as a ward sister, Elizabeth Alsbury (Chapter 13) is able to teach silently, as a role model. Less experienced nurses learn from her through observing her actions rather than being formally taught. Classroom teaching is part of the role for Elizabeth Alsbury, Julie Worth (Chapter 10) and Helen Arrowsmith (Chapter 12). All make contributions to professional education, which gives them a wider sphere of influence not only outside the immediate working environment but also outside the organization.

John Quirk (Chapter 9) demonstrates a different approach through his work with patients who have HIV/AIDS. Patient education depends on sound clinical knowledge and the ability to translate information into forms which the patient can assimilate. Each patient represents a different challenge in this respect because of individual differences in such factors as prior understanding, motivation, intelligence, culture, personality and ability to remember. In John Quirk's field, as in some others, there are the additional factors of unconventional lifestyles and a fear of authority among some patients. In such a context teaching is intended to alter behaviour in order to minimize harm, a strategy which requires active participation on the part of the patient and the willingness of the nurse to negotiate. To achieve this involvement with any learner the specialist practitioner requires (adapted from Meyer, 1987):

- Patience and realism. Change is not easy and those living on the margins of society, whose lives are less organized to begin with, may find it difficult to comply with what is proposed. The same advice may be given over and over again. Kindness and support are essential, especially when people do not succeed in the proposed changes.

- Non-judgemental attitudes. This means accepting people as they are and avoiding condemnation of them, their lifestyle, their management of their illness or any other issue.

- Creativity in devising a variety of approaches which facilitate learning. Individuals have different learning styles. For example, some will benefit from the presentation of factual information backed up by reading material. Others adopt a more reflective approach, watching events to see what happens (Honey, 1988).

- Flexibility and a sense of humour. Not everything will go according to plan. Even the most experienced teacher can find that a carefully prepared class is not what the students really need. The specialist has to be able to adapt to changing situations and to see the funny side of what is happening. If teaching becomes a chore, learning becomes a bore and the intended changes in knowledge, skill or behaviour do not take place.

Monica David's work (Chapter 11) particularly illustrates the importance of these elements. The role of cultural liaison nurse is quite new. It represents part of a drive (Balarajan & Raleigh, 1993) to improve access to health services for members of black and minority ethnic groups because there is a considerable amount of evidence that they are disadvantaged in health care for a number of reasons, including racism (see for example Evers *et al.*, 1988), differing patterns of illness (see for example Raymond & D'Eramo-Melkus, 1993; Haggar, 1994), and culturally determined ideas of health, illness, treatment and care (see for example McAllister & Farquhar, 1992; McGee, 1992) which do not match the dominant, western medical and nursing paradigm. As Monica David points out, it is no use waiting for people, who already feel marginalized, to access services; neither is it acceptable to fall into the trap of believing that, because they do not access them, they neither want nor need them. A particularly common myth is that black and ethnic minority families do not need referral to community agencies because they can cope without them, whereas the truth may be that those agencies are simply not prepared to adapt in order to provide services in a culturally appropriate way (Evers *et al.*, 1988).

One of the important areas of need is that of health promotion and health education. The provision of materials in languages other than English is patchy, and even when available may not be suitable for meeting particular local needs or for overcoming difficulties such as illiteracy. Monica David's account demonstrates some creative ways in which the specialist nurse can engage in effective outreach: through meeting people on their own territory, or using video and audio tape instead of the printed word, and perhaps most importantly by becoming the human face of a faceless organization. People may not know the health authority, but they know the nurse and they can talk to him or her. It is this personal contact which is so important in providing opportunities for misconceptions on both sides to be aired and gradually eroded. This cannot be achieved by one person working alone. As Monica David concludes, the cultural liaison nurse must be part of an overall strategy to achieve change. Managers planning to develop specialist posts need to consider how each post will fit into organizational strategy and how the postholder will be supported in the role.

Researcher

Research activities inform every aspect of the specialist nurse's role, ensuring that practice and teaching are up to date, that innovations are evaluated and that the specialist can act as a resource for others. McGuire and Harwood (1989) propose three levels of research activity which enable all nurses to have some involvement without feeling pressurized into undertaking projects when they do not wish to do so. Similarly there are no rigid rules about who can undertake activity at each level (Dunn, 1991) although it is to be hoped that the specialist nurse will be able to do so.

Level 1 involved developing an awareness of research findings, and reading, evaluating and sharing information with others in order to promote research-based practice. All nurses have some responsibility at this level as part of ensuring that their practice is supported by evidence and keeping abreast of developments in their field. Level 2 involves testing out and applying research findings in practice areas. This could include small scale projects such as Alsbury's (Chapter 13) initial development of the pre-admission clinic. Helen Arrowsmith (Chapter 12) incorporates research-based information into policies and procedures which can be used to ensure good practice even when she is not physically present. She also uses research-based information to help identify needs in practice. Level 3 requires the specialist nurse to be involved in research projects either alone or as a team member, for example Elizabeth Alsbury's evaluation of the pre-admission clinic after three months (Chapter 13).

Conducting research requires particular knowledge, skills and resources (McGee & Notter, 1995), which are usually acquired through higher education. Engaging in research activity at level three requires:

- A sound understanding of the research process plus the ability to think critically and independently
- The ability to ask pertinent questions, and skill in formulating hypotheses
- The ability to plan and carry out ethically responsible projects, drawing on knowledge of sampling, research methods and data analysis
- Skill in obtaining funding and resources for the work
- The ability to express ideas clearly
- A well organized person who is willing to learn from mistakes and who is able to live with uncertainty
- Resources and facilities for publicizing the results (McGee & Notter, 1995; Wabschall, 1987).

Many nurses who take on specialist roles feel unprepared for this aspect of their work and oppressed by the expectations of managers (Arena & Page, 1992). It is important therefore that both parties clarify what is expected and identify training needs for the specialist nurse. Appointment as a specialist should not be regarded as the pinnacle of achievement beyond which no further development is required. It must also be recognized that individuals need time to develop and may not achieve complete mastery of every dimension of the role at the same pace.

Helen Arrowsmith (Chapter 12) and Elizabeth Alsbury (Chapter 13) highlight another dimension allied to the research role. Both these specialist nurses state that they have conducted audits as part of quality monitoring processes. As a matron, Julie Worth (Chapter 10) is responsible for quality assurance in her hospital, undertaking audits and assessing clinical competencies. There are a number of similarities between the research and quality assurance processes (Grant *et al.*, 1991). Research principles complement and can be used to improve quality assurance. In turn a focus on quality can be used to establish a research-based culture among staff who think that research is not for them.

Consultant

The enhanced knowledge and skill enables the specialist nurse to provide advice on a wide range of issues. A single case study by Beyerman (1988) identified four elements of that advice: giving information, making recommendations, questioning and assessment. It is clear that all the specialist nurses in Part 2 maintain a consultant role. Elizabeth Alsbury, in her role as ward sister (Chapter 13), is available to staff who have queries about particular aspects of care. She is able to unite her knowledge of events in theatre with what takes place in the ward and in outpatients to provide a comprehensive picture not available to other staff and thus fulfil all the sub-roles identified by Beyerman. Helen Arrowsmith (Chapter 12) is able to act in a similar way because her role spans hospital settings and patients' homes. Accessibility is immensely important in this consultation role because staff may well not wish to admit that they do not know something or draw attention to their lack of knowledge in any way. Even the act of making an appointment to see the specialist nurse would involve leaving the immediate place of work and would attract attention. Successful consultation provision for staff is therefore very informal and linked in with other work.

John Quirk (Chapter 9) acts as a consultant in a slightly different way. HIV/AIDS patients may choose to access treatment in several centres and in these circumstances the specialist practitioner acts as the linch-pin in maintaining continuity for the patients as well as support and guidance for the staff. This type of consultation requires a specialist to be available over a wide geographical area, usually by telephone, and it may be more cost effective to use this approach than have a heavy involvement in direct care.

Monica David's consultation role is different again (Chapter 11). She adopts a cultural brokerage model which is the 'act of bridging, linking or mediating between groups or persons of differing cultural background for the purpose of reducing conflict or producing change' (Jezewski, 1993). Cultural brokerage involves acting as a bridge between, for example, patients and professionals, the health authority and its customers. Through her networking among local groups, Monica David has become able to act as broker between the black and minority ethnic groups and the health authority. Inevitably these are situations of unequal power and the broker's remit is to function as mediator, interpreting each party's wishes to the other until understanding is achieved. In doing so Monica David alerts those involved to the miscommunication that can occur. A nod and a smile do not always mean agreement or even that the person has understood. Assumptions and stereotypes have to be challenged in a constructive way if culturally competent services are to be developed (McGee, 1994).

Finally, Julie Worth's consultation role is for the organization as a whole (Chapter 10). As matron she is responsible for identifying areas of risk either in practice or in the hospital environment generally. In some instances she can effect change herself but in others she may have to advise the organization about actions required. Evidence suggests that one of the advantages of employing specialist nurses is that, as identified individuals, they can advise the health care organization at the most senior levels. Managing such an organization is an extremely complex task and senior personnel cannot be expected to know in detail about every aspect of service provision. In this context, the advice of a specialist nurse is invaluable (McGee *et al.*, 1996).

Leader and manager

Leadership may be defined as influencing individuals or groups towards the achievement of goals (Gournic, 1989). Leadership is not coercive but does involve giving directions about and towards an end point (Al-Kandari, 1993). Leaders are characterized by a willingness to innovate and experiment. They habitually challenge the accepted view of the world, question routines and are not afraid to make changes. Moreover, they encourage others to do the same. Secondly, they have a vision of what they want to achieve and will actively recruit others to their cause, fostering cooperative styles of working in order to achieve their aims, and rewarding their achievements. They inspire others through their actions and can remain level-headed in a crisis (Al-Kandari, 1993). They have well-developed communication skills, and a 'leadership language' (Dillard, 1993) which is used to support and encourage others.

John Quirk (Chapter 9) draws attention to the power of leaders to effect change. Nurses who took up the challenge of HIV/AIDS nursing were trailblazing a new area of practice. They were leading both professionals and the public in combating fear, ignorance and prejudice through a reappraisal of accepted opinions about sexuality and lifestyle. Through this they were able to develop nursing knowledge and practice, providing leadership for nurses in a variety of care settings.

Management differs from leadership in terms of its focus. It is essentially the art of achieving organizational goals through working with individuals and groups (Simons, 1993). A manager is given authority by the organization to set objectives commensurate with the organizational goals and to develop, direct and monitor staff in the achievement of those objectives (Gournic, 1989).

In reality, leadership and management are intertwined. Leadership needs good organizational skills and the authority to direct people when necessary. Management requires leadership as part of motiving and developing staff. Julie Worth's account of her role as matron in an independent hospital (Chapter 10) provides an interesting example of the integration of the two. She describes the managerial strategies, such as the development and direction of staff through the IPR process and further professional education, and the quality assurance strategy. However, she is also aware of using well-developed communication skills. More importantly, she has a pivotal role in effecting change, providing both leadership and the management tools with which to accomplish what is required.

Conclusion

It is evident from this discussion that the specialist nursing role is multi-dimensional. While a number of separate elements can be identified, in reality they overlap and inform one another. Expert care is impossible without a sound knowledge of research findings, but that care in turn provides ideas for future research work. Leadership skills are essential in enabling the nurse to act as a change agent, but unless that nurse is a first class, research-based practitioner, change may well not be for the better. Teaching is dependent on both clinical practice and research, plus the advanced communication skills required for leadership and management.

Separating the various elements of the specialist practice role is useful in trying to understand the broad parameters of this form of practice, but it may be that in doing so we lose sight of the integrated whole. It is unlikely that any specialist nurse ever says, 'Now I am teaching, later I will be leading and tomorrow I will be researching'. The integrated nature of the specialist role means that at least some of these activities are taking place simultaneously without conscious awareness that they can be labelled as different. Specialist practice must be regarded as a single entity, but each practitioner has different strengths and develops the role in a way which suits both them and their employers. It may be that this freedom is an essential ingredient in making such roles successful.

References

Al-Kandari, F. (1993) Personality styles. In: *Transformational Leadership in Nursing* (ed. A. Marriner-Twomey). Mosby Yearbook, St Louis.

Arena, D. & Page, N. (1992) The imposter phenomenon in the CNS role. *Image Journal of Nursing Scholarship*, **24** (2), 121–5.

Balarajan, R. & Raleigh, V.S. (1993) *Ethnicity and Health: a Guide for the NHS*. Department of Health, London.

Benner, P. (1984) *From Novice to Expert: Excellence and Power in Clinical Nursing Practice*. Addison-Wesley, Menlo Park.

Beyerman, K. (1988) Consultation roles of the clinical nurse specialist: a case study. *Clinical Nurse Specialist*, **2** (2), 91–5.

Dillard, N. (1993) Development of hardiness. In: *Transformational Leadership in Nursing* (ed. A. Marriner-Twomey). Mosby Yearbook, St Louis.

Dreyfus, H. & Dreyfus, S. (1996) The relationship of theory and practice in the acquisition of skill. In: *Expertise in Nursing Practice. Caring, Clinical Judgement and Ethics* (eds P. Benner, C. Tanner & C. Chesla). Springer Publishing Company, New York.

Dunn, B. (1991) Who should do research in nursing? *Professional Nurse*, January, 190–6.

Evers, H., Cameron, E., Badger, F. & Atkin, K. (1988) *Community Care Working Papers, No. 11*. Department of Social Medicine, University of Birmingham.

Girard, N. (1987) The CNS: development of the role. In: *The Clinical Nurse Specialist. Perspectives on Practice* (ed. S. Menard). John Wiley and Sons, New York.

Gournic, J. (1989) Clinical leadership, management and the CNS. In: *The Clinical Nurse Specialist in Theory and Practice* (eds A. Hamric & J. Spross), 2nd edn. W.B. Saunders, Philadelphia.

Grant, M., Fleming, I. & Calvanico, A. (1991) Research and quality assurance. In: *Conducting and Using Nursing Research in the Clinical Setting* (eds M. Mate & K.T. Kirchoff). Williams and Wilkins, Baltimore.

Haggar, V. (1994) Cultural challenge. *Nursing Times*, 13 April, **90** (15), 71–2.

Heffline, M. (1992) Establishing the role of the clinical nurse specialist in post-anaesthesia care. *Journal of Post Anaesthesia Nursing*, **17** (5), 305–11.

Honey, P. (1988) You are what you learn. *Nursing Times*, 7 September, **84** (36), 34, 36.

Jezewski, M. (1993) Culture brokering as a model for advocacy. *Nursing and Health Care*, **14** (2), 78–85.

Koetters, T. (1989) Clinical practice and direct patient care. In: *The Clinical Nurse Specialist in Theory and Practice* (eds A. Hamric & J. Spross), 2nd edn. W.B. Saunders, Philadelphia.

McAllister, G. & Farquhar, M. (1992) Health beliefs: a cultural division? *Journal of Advanced Nursing*, 17, 1447–54.

McGee, P. (1992) *Teaching Transcultural Care. A Guide for Teachers of Nursing and Health Care*. Chapman and Hall, London.

McGee, P. (1994) Culturally sensitive and culturally comprehensive care. *British Journal of Nursing*, **3** (15), 789–92.

McGee, P., Castledine, G. & Brown, B. (1996) *A survey of specialist and advanced practice in England*. Report published by the Nursing Research Unit, University of Central England, Birmingham.

McGee, P. & Notter, J. (1995) *Research Appreciation: an Initial Guide for Nurses and Health Care Professionals.* Quay Books, Nr Dinton, Salisbury.

McGuire, D. & Harwood, K. (1989) The CNS as researcher. In: *The Clinical Nurse Specialist in Theory and Practice* (eds A. Hamric & J. Spross), 2nd edn. W.B. Saunders, Philadelphia.

Menard, S. (1987) The CNS as practitioner. In: *The Clinical Nurse Specialist. Perspectives on Practice* (ed. S. Menard). John Wiley and Sons, New York.

Meyer, J. (1987) The CNS as teacher. In: *The Clinical Nurse Specialist. Perspectives on Practice* (ed. S. Menard). John Wiley and Sons, New York.

Raymond, N. & D'Eramo-Melkus, G. (1993) Non-insulin-dependent diabetes and obesity in the black and hispanic population: culturally sensitive management. *Diabetes Education*, Jul–Aug, **19** (4), 313–7.

Simons, M. (1993) Changing visions, the history of leadership. In: *Transformational Leadership in Nursing*, (ed. A. Marriner-Twomey). Mosby Yearbook, St Louis.

The Nuffield Provincial Hospitals Trust (1954) *The work of nurses in hospital wards.* Report of a job analysis. The Nuffield Provincial Hospitals Trust, London.

UKCC (1994) *The Future of Professional Practice – the Council's Standards for Education and Practice Following Registration.* United Kingdom Central Council for Nursing, Midwifery and Health Visiting, London.

Wabschall, J. (1987) The CNS as researcher. In: *The Clinical Nurse Specialist. Perspectives on Practice*, (ed. S. Menard). John Wiley and Sons, New York.

Chapter 9

Specialist Practice in HIV/AIDS Nursing

John Quirk

To many people who work in nursing the role of a specialist or advanced nursing practitioner is little understood. We are often seen as aloof and remote from the day to day business of providing hands-on nursing care. In providing a nursing service at a higher level or on a wider scale we may attract the suspicion and mistrust of the very colleagues we aim to empower, support and enable.

What makes a nurse a specialist nurse? First, there must be an identified group of patients who require a service specifically aimed at meeting a demand or need, in my case patients with HIV infection and AIDS. The AIDS epidemic has provided a challenge to science, medicine and society and has seen the development of a group of nurses who have had to adapt their work practice to provide appropriate care for a group of patients stigmatized and marginalized by society. Nurses who took up this challenge in the early 1980s did so in an atmosphere of fear, ignorance and rejection.

As Wright pointed out in Faugier & Hicken (1996):

> 'Many nurses approached this new health challenge positively, and shared the potential to be at the leading edge of humanitarian caring, others became bogged down by ignorance and prejudice.'

The nursing specialism of HIV/AIDS had its catalyst in the 'setting up of specialist units and nursing roles, training courses, conferences and reports' and so helped to diminish many problems by building awareness among nurses about the realities of AIDS (Faugier & Hicken, 1996). Twenty years on much has changed in how we treat and care for patients with HIV and AIDS, but sadly elements of ignorance and intolerance are still with us today.

Nurses who embarked on this road played an active and important part in the creation of an environment where patients could be cared for in an atmosphere of tolerance and acceptance. This innovative process of establishing a specialist service could not have taken place if nurses involved in HIV/AIDS care had not challenged existing nursing practice, attitudes and managerial structures. The reward for nurses involved in this formative period was the realization of the potential of the nursing role as a responsive agent to changing patient care needs.

Specialist practice in the field of HIV/AIDS care challenges nurses on many levels. It may force us to examine our own sexuality and attitudes to the sexual practices of others. Our patients may lead lifestyles very different from our own or incredibly similar. Prejudice within society and the nursing and medical professions brought about one of the first organizations in Britain that dealt with the AIDS epidemic: 'The Terence Higgins Trust in 1983 was one of the first national voluntary organizations to respond to all aspects of the AIDS and HIV health crisis' (NAM, 1997a). One of these aspects was poor nursing care brought about through ignorance, prejudice and fear.

An honest examination of our own prejudices and fears is needed before we can attempt to provide sensitive and holistic care to our patients. The art and science of nursing decrees that all our patients, from whatever lifestyle or background, receive the same standard of care.

The argument for specialist nurses in HIV/AIDS

A decision to work in the field of HIV/AIDS care is viewed as an odd choice by some nurses and elements of society. To enable us to care for patients living with HIV and AIDS we have to align ourselves with a group of people who often inhabit the margins of society. To provide an appropriate standard of care for these patients we must have assessed their 'needs' appropriately. One example of this is by researching the practice and opinions of others who work in the field. The nurse specialist may choose to adapt a model of care carried out elsewhere to suit his or her own needs locally. In the early days of the epidemic the adaptation of the palliative care model of care was appropriate for large numbers of patients dying of AIDS. However this model of care does not meet all the needs of people living with HIV infection on a clinical, social and personal basis.

Alternatively the specialist nurse may embark on a self directed process that examines in depth the needs of the patients/clients to be served. The level and type of knowledge gained places the specialist nurse in a position where advanced practice can be achieved. The tools used may be in the form of audit, research or a broad 'needs analysis' involving discussion and consultation with other health, statutory and voluntary carers. To ensure that our knowledge base remains current and effective a monitoring or review process must then be set up. Multi-disciplinary and peer review is an important factor in keeping our practice relevant to the needs of our patients. Strategies must be formulated whereby this knowledge and insight is shared with our nursing colleagues and other members of the multi disciplinary team. No one nurse or practitioner can provide for all the needs of a patient. Clear and efficient lines of communication enable the specialist nurse to work as a vital component in an HIV/AIDS care team.

The knowledge base in specialist care of HIV/AIDS patients

The type of knowledge demanded will vary greatly depending on the setting in which we provide our care. Nurses working in an acute setting are very much removed from the everyday environment and problems of their patients. An HIV patient who is an injecting drug user may conform to the rules and regulations of a hospital ward during a period of treatment. However upon discharge into their 'normal' environment, individuals revert to unsafe and unhygienic injecting practice. A specialist nurse with an insight into the lifestyle and behaviour of his/her patients outside the institutional setting can negotiate harm reduction strategies to conserve veins and avoid infection. Through discussion and negotiation a clean vein may be left intact to enable venous access for blood testing. This type of behaviour modification programme benefits the patient and enhances the role of the nurse. The nurse, through an expanded knowledge base, is able to influence a patient's behaviour outside the acute setting, thus achieving a therapeutic partnership with the patient.

The nurse involved in this process may have developed the knowledge needed through previous work experience or may have embarked on a concerted learning process of reading, discussion and listening to the problems encountered by the patient. The end result is a nurse whose practice has been adapted to provide a better and more appropriate type of care for the patient.

The experience of any nurse, including the HIV specialist nurse working in the community, is vastly different from the hospital setting. The protection of the institution and the immediate support of other health carers is removed. The community based nurse must function in a setting where the patient is in their 'normal' environment and the nurse is the embodiment of the health service.

In this setting the specialist nurse takes on the role of a health care 'care manager', identifying the needs of patients, partners, families and carers. Recognition of the patients' personal beliefs, cultural background and previous life experiences all have a bearing on the type and level of communication experienced. An example of this are HIV/AIDS patients from sub-Saharan Africa who have been traumatized by war, rape and intimidation. The refugee with a fear and distrust of authority may need time to build up a level of trust in a nurse or care worker. A community setting is seen to be more conducive to this process as it occurs in the patient's home and not in the unfamiliar institutional setting of a hospital.

HIV/AIDS patients generally receive treatment and support via an outpatients/genito-urinary medicine clinic. HIV/AIDS specialist nurses represent a link between the centres of excellence and the community. HIV infected people may choose to access services in their local area or travel to genito-urinary medicine clinics and outpatient departments attached to the larger teaching hospitals. This element of choice increases the demands on the nurse specialist caring for these patients. Liaison and communication must often take place between more than one treatment centre, requiring the specialist nurse to raise their profile in clinics and departments out of their designated work area. This requires the specialist nurse to have a greater degree of autonomy and flexibility to facilitate liaison with a number of institutions and organizations providing care for HIV/AIDS patients.

This situation has the potential for co-operation as well as conflict, especially when the specialist nurse highlights deficiencies in service provision. An example of this is where a patient's medication needs may be met by a treatment centre while their dietary needs are ignored. Patient compliance with a new and complex treatment regime can be improved when a nurse specialist assesses a need for simpler or clearer explanation of drugs and their action. Timely and responsive feedback to the treatment centre can avoid a breakdown in communication between the patient and their doctor.

Observing the way our patients live in a home setting often makes us aware of their non-health care needs. The provision of health care is linked with other factors such as housing, benefits, alternative lifestyles, recreational drug use and so many factors clearly not traditionally within a health care remit. We are forced to look at the needs of our patients on a wider scale. We take on the role of a patient advocate in areas that are not the traditional or expected remit of nurses. Advocacy brings with it the need for the specialist nurse to have the ability to articulate for the patient that which they need. An understanding of how and where these needs can be met sets the specialist nurse apart.

Research and evaluation of specialist practice

A nurse specialist providing a flexible and responsive service in a community setting has the potential to improve the quality of life and the quality of health care of the patients in their care. The quality of health care is enhanced in a number of ways, including:

- Prevention of unnecessary re-admission to hospital
- Augmentation of the role of the general practitioner
- Acting as a resource to other nursing and health care staff both in hospital and the community

Research concerning the advanced practice roles of clinical nurse specialists, nurse practitioners and nurse midwives has not only provided emerging models of care but also validated the effectiveness of nurses in the care and management of HIV infected individuals. Clinical nurse specialists have demonstrated flexibility in role functions by serving as direct care providers, consultants and care managers in both inpatient and community based settings (Layzell & McCarthy, 1993; McCann, 1991; Sherman & Johnson, 1991). Ongoing research and audit into care outcomes and factors that influence quality of life give rise to improved practice, thus reinforcing the value of the specialist nurse providing care at an enhanced level. Audit of the nature of our interaction with our medical or nursing colleagues is a useful tool in ascertaining the attitudes of fellow professionals to our role.

Working as a specialist nurse

To adequately meet the needs of a diverse and varied patient group the nurse specialist must be able to provide a flexible and responsive service. Table 9.1 shows the basis of a structure in which a specialist nurse can function.

As nurses we must recognize that patients respond best to medical and nursing intervention when they feel they have control over what happens to them. Knowledge enables informed consent which implies control. Ruth Sims and Veronica Moss of London's Mildmay Mission Hospital, while examining the palliative care needs of people with AIDS, highlight the benefit for patients of greater control for both patient and nurse when they comment:

'In order to give patients control it is necessary for nurses to be given a greater degree of freedom and flexibility within the structure in which they work so as not to be bound by routine or rigid timetables. It will be necessary to ensure that managers understand the philosophy for nursing care so that inflexibility on their part does not restrict practice.' (Sims & Moss, 1995)

Change is a constant aspect of our lives, and some choose to resist or work against it. As nurses we must not fear that which is necessary to improve patient care or worry that we may reduce our standing as essential elements of the health care team. We must seize the opportunity that specialist

Table 9.1   The basic structure in which an HIV/AIDS specialist nurse can function.

(1)   A working environment that enables the specialist nurse to deliver a high standard of research and evidence based care to patients with HIV/AIDS.

(2)   The ability to visit and assess appropriately referred patients in a setting that is conducive to the free and confidential exchange of information and knowledge.

(3)   A relevant and mutually negotiated job description with built-in review and monitoring structures and timetables.

(4)   Psychological and clinical supervision from appropriate professional sources to provide feedback, guidance and recognition of the achievement of goals and professional growth.

(5)   The provision of a management framework within which the specialist nurse can function as a specialist practitioner meeting the recognized needs of a group of patients. To work within accepted professional boundaries in a flexible and responsive manner.

(6)   Participation within appropriate audit and research programmes evaluating the effectiveness of service provision to our patients. Development of self generated research programmes into care outcomes.

(7)   To educate other health care, statutory, voluntary staff and service users as to the role and purpose of the specialist nurse or advanced practitioner.

(8)   We have a duty to ourselves, our patients and our nursing and medical colleagues to maintain our skills, knowledge and identity as nurses. In doing so we enhance the standing of our profession and ensure that it unceasingly achieves its goal of providing appropriate standards of care to our patients.

(9)   Ongoing self directed education and update programmes on the changing needs of people living with HIV/AIDS. The negotiation of budgetary allocation to enable the specialist nurse to function as a health care 'care manager'.

nursing practice presents. In doing so we enhance the role of the nurse as an agent of change, reviewer of care provision and advocate for those in our care and thus achieve growth on a personal and professional level.

HIV/AIDS specialism and the future

The future of the specialism of HIV/AIDS nursing is fluid and one in which the politics of envy play a part. Many in government, medicine and society see our specialty as having had too much money for far too long. Ring-fenced monies are no longer protected and the level of service that has proved effective in meeting the needs of patients with HIV/AIDS will be diminished. My reply to those who criticize the amount of money spent on AIDS treatment and HIV prevention is to point out that the UK has one of the lowest ratios of HIV infection per capita in Europe.

As the National AIDS Reference Manual points out, 'France has already reported more cases of AIDS in the Paris region alone than in the whole of the UK'. The incidence of AIDS per million people was more than three times greater in France in 1994 than in the UK. The worst affected European country is Spain, with an incidence of 156 AIDS cases per million in 1994 (NAM, 1997b).

We only need look at the reaction of countries such as France and Spain to realize that the early recognition of the threat and a concerted response to it enabled the UK to reduce the impact of the AIDS epidemic. Nurses have benefited from being part of the social and health care response. The UK's response to the HIV/AIDS epidemic has proved the worth of concerted and co-ordinated HIV prevention campaigns. Attention was focused on our infection control practices, attitudes to blood borne infections such as hepatitis B and C and the way we react to patients in our care. Stigma is a word seldom used by nurses and health care staff; however, HIV/AIDS has forced us to recognize the way in which society in general and health carers label and stigmatize those whom we have a duty to care for. To work with a patient who is HIV positive is to work with someone whom society is all too ready to label and stigmatize. Cultural, ethnic, immigration and sexual issues all combine to provide a challenge to the nurse who seeks to meet the health care needs of HIV/AIDS patients.

Just as the pattern of the epidemic has changed and is changing so does the way we treat its manifestations. Palliative care was once considered the ideal specialty for the HIV/AIDS nurse specialist. More recently it has been argued that virology is a suitable place for HIV/AIDS to be classified, along with hepatitis B and C. Sexual health and HIV are linked by the fact that the majority of HIV infection is transmitted sexually. There are some who would like to see the speciality of HIV/AIDS nursing wound down or subsumed into a more traditional specialty; however, it should be evident to clear thinking health care professionals that specialist HIV/AIDS nurses will continue to adapt to the varied and changing needs of people with HIV infection and AIDS.

Recognition of, and the provision of a framework within which nurses have evolved to a specialist level, are basic requirements for the future of specialist nurses in HIV/AIDS care. The AIDS epidemic will not go away, nor will the nurses who have chosen to work in this area of nursing.

References

Faugier, J. & Hicken, I. (1996) *AIDS and HIV – The Nursing Responses*, p. 50. Chapman and Hall, London.

Layzell, S. & McCarthy, M. (1993) Specialist or generic community nursing care for HIV/AIDS patients? *Journal of Advanced Nursing*, **18** (4), 531–7.

McCann, K. (1991) The work of the specialist AIDS home support team: the views and experience of patients using the service. *Journal of Advanced Nursing Practice*, **16** (7), 832–83.

NAM (1997a) National AIDS Manual, UK AIDS Directory, p. 186. NAM Publications, London.

NAM (1997b) National AIDS Manual, UK AIDS Reference Manual, p. 76. NAM Publications, London.

Sherman, J.J. & Johnson, P.K. (1991) Nursing care management. *Quality Assurance and Utilization Review*, **6** (4), 142–5.

Sims, R. & Moss, V. (1995) *Palliative Care for People with AIDS*, p. 31. Edward Arnold, London.

Chapter 10

A Descriptive Account of the Role of the Matron at an Independent Hospital

Julie Worth

Nuffield Hospitals is a charitable organization, established in 1947. Today Nuffield Hospitals is one of the largest group of independent hospitals consisting of 39 hospitals across England and Scotland. The Nuffield Hospital where I am employed as the matron provides independent health care services for an overall catchment population of 475 000 people.

The independent health care services which have been developed at the hospital include a wide variety of diagnostic and treatment facilities available on an outpatient or inpatient basis. The outpatient services include: diagnostic imaging and interventional radiology, bone densitometry, MRI and spiral CT. There is a fully equipped pathology department, physiotherapy department, health screening service and a minor procedures clinic. There are five consulting rooms covering all general medical and surgical specialties. The 45 *en suite* bedrooms accommodate patients undergoing a wide range of medical and surgical interventions on an inpatient and day-care basis.

The role of the matron

The matron is accountable to the hospital manager. She is a member of the senior management team which includes the hospital manager, business office manager, marketing manager and hotel services manager. The matron provides clinical information and advice when major strategic decisions are being made by the hospital manager and senior management. The matron, along with other members of the senior management team, attends medical advisory committee meetings. The medical advisory committee is an elected representative body of the hospital consultant users and local general practitioners.

154

The hospital is registered with the local health authority. The matron is the named person with the health authority who is accountable for ensuring that commonly agreed standards of care are implemented.

Risk management

The matron is accountable for clinical risk management within the hospital and must investigate all accident reports, incident reports and complaints fully. By testing out current risk management systems that are in place, revising and replacing them as necessary, he/she will ensure that the hospital meets all its legal obligations. As part of the risk management role, the matron co-ordinates the statutory audit and assessment requirements which the hospital undertakes.

The matron is responsible for ensuring that all mandatory lectures are undertaken by hospital staff to comply with risk management, including manual handling, cardiac pulmonary resuscitation and infection control regulations.

Management of resources

The matron works closely with the business office manager to establish the clinical budgets within the hospital business plan. Once the clinical budgets have been agreed with the hospital manager the matron is responsible for ensuring that all expenditure within the clinical departments remains within the agreed budget. This budget includes staffing costs for each clinical department, expenditure on equipment through the minor capital budget, consumables usage and recapture of costs by ensuring patients are charged for consumables appropriately.

Quality assurance strategy

The matron is responsible for establishing and implementing the hospital's quality assurance strategy, to ensure customer expectations of their clinical care are exceeded. This is achieved through an ongoing programme of standard setting, auditing practice against set standards, reviewing the standards against the findings and implementing the changes.

Independent hospitals have to ensure that all their customer needs are addressed. While the matron must monitor patients' (who attend for health screening) requirements, she must also ensure that the consultant users' needs are met. An important method of discovering customer requirements is through close communication with patients, clients and consultants, to discover on a personal basis how they perceive the hospital's services and how improvements can be made. Another method is through customer questionnaire surveys. The matron and the senior management team analyse and interpret the findings before making improvements to customer services. Each hospital employee has access to the customer questionnaire responses and can make suggestions for improvement through focus groups and departmental meetings. This ensures that staff can initiate changes and have an understanding of the need for change in various hospital practices.

Professional development

The matron is responsible for co-ordinating external quality audit programmes throughout the hospital, for example, Kings Fund Organisational Audit. Private medical insurance companies frequently request evidence of quality programmes that are in place. The matron plays a major role in communicating these programmes to them.

Each registered nurse within Nuffield Hospitals has a performance standard portfolio which is focused on the nurse's level of knowledge and skill performance against a given set of criteria. This skill assessment enables each registered nurse to develop a clear understanding of their own professional development needs. The matron then aligns professional education and skill development in conjunction with the hospital business plan's objectives. For example, if a new service is being developed within the hospital, such as a high dependency unit or diabetic clinic, the matron must be able to deliver the clinical skills to support such a development.

The matron promotes the development of networks not only among other Nuffield Hospitals but also with local NHS Trust hospitals, where staff with specialist interests have opportunities to work alongside their colleagues in other hospitals to develop their nursing competencies further. The matron co-ordinates the individual performance review programme which is undertaken annually. The performance standards can be used to identify personal objectives for each member of the nursing staff. The matron must also ensure that her own professional development is addressed. This is achieved by attending pertinent conferences and postgraduate diploma courses.

The matron plays a major role in supporting further education and training for staff, by ensuring staff have access to library facilities, to a wide range of current clinical journals and to local college/university courses, together with access to the Nuffield Hospitals' Education Centre. The matron may hold seminars for staff or invite outside speakers to address the clinical staff.

Communication

It is crucial to the whole organization that the matron is an effective communicator. They can achieve this through establishing formal meetings which are minuted. These minutes are kept in each department for staff to read. For effective two way communication to take place, the matron must talk to individual members of staff within their departments and when necessary be a good listener. The matron must also employ compassionate counselling skills, and on other occasions skills of diplomacy. Within the counselling framework the matron can monitor and evaluate professional practices.

Management of change

A major part of the matron's role is to instigate and develop change within all aspects of clinical practice. The matron must be aware of changes within the market place and implement changes accordingly, for example managed care and clinical care pathways which are founded on evidence-based practice.

The development of new private medical insurance company agreements with hospital groups, for example partnership agreements, means that the matron has to be involved with medical insurance companies and work closely with the business office of the hospital, in order to ensure that the insurance company will fund the patient's treatment.

Conclusion

The matron's role encompasses a wide range of responsibilities. The most important area is the quality of care given to all the hospital's customers. This is achieved by establishing effective risk management systems, performance standards for nurses, and effective education and training for clinical and non-clinical staff, auditing customers' expectations and perceptions in conjunction with auditing professional practice.

The matron's role within the development and implementation of the hospital business plan is crucial in achieving budgetary targets and planned developments.

Matrons achieve their own and the hospital's objectives by influencing the change and managing the transition, evaluating the activity and giving appropriate feedback to the relevant groups, before commencing the process again.

Chapter 11
Cultural Awareness and Customer Care

Monica David

What is the difference between customer care and cultural awareness? Perhaps if we say customer care of the individual that would lead into addressing the cultural issues of each client and stop assumptions that clients from black and minority ethnic backgrounds such as Sikh, Chinese, Muslim or Rastafarian will automatically do things in a certain way. If we ask, 'What are your individual needs and how can we work together to meet those needs?' we have a two-way learning process which is beneficial to both professionals and clients.

Why do we need cultural liaison officers?

My role as cultural liaison officer, public health medicine department, is very important because it looks at black and minority ethnic health issues from both sides, the client and the health authority. The main areas of concern focus on primary care issues.

Communication

There are two main issues here. First, many ethnic minority adults do not speak English and rely on friends or family members to interpret for them, which poses questions of confidentiality. There is major concern about the use of children for interpreting purposes, e.g. the child's ability to tell the parent what the doctor has said and what it means. How do we know what the child has said? What is the parent's understanding of what the child or the doctor has said, and what a burden to lay on a child to maybe have to tell a parent they have a serious illness? There is a need for health trained interpreters and link workers, with training for professionals on how to access interpreter and link worker services and work alongside them.

Secondly, most black and minority ethnic people will not ask a doctor questions because they feel the doctor knows best and whatever they say must be right. Also, their knowledge of health issues can be very limited and they would possibly not have the ability to question; so when asked if they understand they will nod and say 'yes' but do not really know what is happening. It is often assumed, for example, that African Caribbeans have understood the doctor because they speak English. This is not so as English is often spoken with a dialect, e.g. patois, and cultural beliefs are different. They do not want to look foolish by saying, 'I don't understand you'.

Availability and appropriateness of services

Access to services and information which are culturally sensitive is essential. Lack of understanding of GP (General Practitioner) services and how to use them can cause confusion for many black and minority ethnic people and can lead to an overuse of the service in some cases. There is a need for basic leaflets or audio cassettes in different languages with information on GP services, e.g. appointment systems, how to take medication, use of the pharmacist for treatment of minor illnesses like coughs and colds, and practice staff information. This information could then be discussed within the home or community centre or at health education sessions within the doctor's surgery.

I work closely with our minority ethnic health advisor in health promotion to promote access to services and healthy lifestyles through properly targeted, non-jargonistic information and training, e.g. in relation to coronary hearth disease. Even though there is a high incidence of coronary heart disease among black and minority ethnic people, there is very little understanding of the illness so it makes no sense to translate coronary heart disease leaflets into all languages and say 'Here, read this'. Some cannot read their own language, and even if they can, their level of understanding may be limited.

Therefore the health promotion advisor and myself work together to arrange specific coronary heart disease awareness sessions in a place in which black and minority ethnic people feel comfortable, e.g. Ghudwara, temple, or community centre. For example, if the clients are Punjabi speaking, we show a video on coronary heart disease in Punjabi and bring in interpreters to that questions can be asked and answered. Audio cassettes are much more effective than leaflets because even if there are language and reading barriers, the spoken word will be better understood if it is in the appropriate language and dialect. In these sessions we would also involve the community dietician to give advice on healthy eating using Asian foods – foods that people can relate to, for example, the use of wholemeal flour for roti and chapati, or how to cook without or use less ghee. We give advice on exercise programmes that are culturally sensitive, and use the media, e.g. Asian radio and Asian Talking Newspapers, to help promote a healthy lifestyle and 'look after your heart' positive messages. This is just one example of how we can work together to raise awareness of health issues that affect black and minority ethnic communities.

I have met with nearly all the agencies within the borough where I work with a view to looking at service provision. Some were apprehensive at the beginning because talk of culture means 'how much will it cost?' Comments like, 'We have tried approaching the communities but with very little success', and 'We don't feel there is anything else we can do' were quite common. Then I would say, 'OK, let's look at things differently, not in a "them and us" situation but working together to look at differences and how both can be accommodated. I am a black and minority ethnic person, has it been difficult talking to me?'

Assumptions and prejudices can be talked about and addressed. Now these same agencies are liaising with members of the black and minority ethnic communities to promote their services. Black and minority ethnic issues are being addressed at their meetings and on the agenda of their steering groups. I attend meetings, sit on committees, give presentations and foster a network in which people work together, acknowledging different cultures and backgrounds and promoting health care services to address their specific health needs for all, not just the majority. This work can only be done by networking with other agencies, often outside the borough, seeing what is being done elsewhere, asking advice and working with the ground workers who work directly with the community on a day to day basis.

My work within public health is then carried on by a community based cultural liaison officer working directly with the communities to raise awareness. In hospital, services are covered by a hospital based cultural liaison officer who provides cultural awareness for hospital staff with regard to issues such as diet, religious beliefs, death and bereavement. The four workers in the minority ethnic health team (three cultural liaison officers and one health promotion adviser) meet on a regular basis to discuss issues and to structure health care to meet the needs.

My role is also essential in a training and advisory capacity for other professionals in order to change beliefs and attitudes. Some of the statements I commonly hear are:

(1) 'Well, we provide the service, but the black and minority ethnic groups don't come; we've sent out leaflets and questionnaires but they have not replied so we assume that they don't need our services.'

My response to this is: are we saying that black and minority ethnic people don't get sick? If they are not coming to you, where are they going – or are they suffering in silence? Ask yourself why black and minority ethnic people don't access your service. Do they know of your services? Do you want them to know of your services? What does your service say about your organization; is it seen as, or portrayed as, a white service, e.g. look at your staffing, surroundings, literature and terminology.

- What is your and your staff's understanding of different cultures and backgrounds?
- When the people do come what is your attitude towards them?
- Who do you talk to about your service and how leaflets are not effective if the portrayal and terminology are wrong?

(2) 'Well, they are looked after by their families aren't they, so that's why they don't need us.'

My response to this is: the extended family is a myth. It is not the same as 'back home' we look after our own. The economic climate plays a big part in the family structure – unemployment, bad housing, working away from home and differences in attitude between young and old. Look at the minority ethnic elders who are now starting to enter nursing homes.

(3) 'We don't have a problem, we treat everyone the same!'

My response to this is that treating everyone the same can mean a number of things:

- The blinkered approach – 'I don't want to see a difference or talk about it'
- The 'I'm the way I am and they can take me as they find me' approach, which can be offensive to everyone
- 'I am polite and treat everybody with whom I come into contact with respect'

The last one is much easier to work with because respect for others can break down barriers on its own. Black and minority ethnic people feel comfortable with that; it is often the unspoken word and body language with attitude that causes offence.

In effect what I am saying is, 'Let's look at your service provision from another angle; often how you portray yourself is seen as stereotypical and the reason or one of the reasons that black and minority ethnic people don't come.'

Conclusion

Cultural liaison work is difficult but can be very rewarding when you see agencies who have said, 'We realize there is a problem but we don't know how to address it', then start to move forward and actually want to continue discussion and look at differences and try to work alongside you to bring about change.

The communities for so long have felt that things will never change, and there is still a long way to go. Some stereotypical attitudes will never change completely. In my opinion everyone has a certain amount of like and dislike; it is when you inflict them on another person that it becomes a problem.

The health service is a caring service for all people and should be seen as such. To fulfil the criteria for cultural liaison work, it is necessary to employ people from the black and minority ethnic communities on permanent contracts as the work is ongoing with the need to build confidence on both sides. There needs to be commitment from the health authority to bring about change, and the postholder needs the full support of line managers and senior managers. Minority ethnic health should not be an added extra but part of mainstream funding. We need to stop carrying out little projects which are costly and have little or no effect, and start thinking about long term lasting health provision for all.

Chapter 12
The Nutrition Nurse Specialist

Helen Arrowsmith

Introduction

The role of the nutrition nurse specialist (NNS) has developed over recent years and there are approximately 62 nutrition nurse specialists recorded as members of the national nurses nutrition group. This group is an advisory and support group for the NNS and general nurses with an interest in nutrition, prevention of malnutrition and provision of nutritional support. Its function is to keep the members updated with current issues, practice and innovations in audit and research.

The NNS usually practises independently but most will also work as part of a multi disciplinary team. At Birmingham Heartlands Hospital the nutrition team consists of the following members, whose collaboration will be discussed later:

- Consultant in gastroenterology
- Senior registrar/lecturer and registrar in gastroenterology
- Senior dietitian
- Nutrition nurse specialist
- Pharmacist (aseptic services)
- Clinical biochemist

The national nurse nutrition group is a founder group of the British Association of Parenteral and Enteral Nutrition, a national group consisting of founder groups of the other disciplines mentioned above, including a patient support group. Parenteral and enteral describe the route by which nutrition is given to the patient, parenteral meaning nutrition given by a route other than the gut, i.e. the venous route, and enteral pertaining to the delivery of nutrition into the gut. The founder groups work closely together as part of the British Association of Parenteral and Enteral Nutrition in raising national awareness of the nutritional needs of the patient, identifying disease-related malnutrition and offering advice and education on the provision of nutritional support by means of multi-disciplinary conference, sharing research findings, formal education and the provision of national guidelines. As secretary to the national nurses nutrition group from December 1995 to 1997 I believe it is important for specialist nurses to have a forum such as this to provide peer support, motivate and promote a high standard of nursing care.

My current title as an NNS is 'clinical nurse specialist nutrition'. Although I refer to nutrition nurse specialist here, titles may vary depending on the hospital, seniority, grade or qualifications of the nurse, particularly if there is more than one NNS in a team. The ultimate aim of my service is to identify patients who require nutritional support and enhance their quality of care.

The British Association of Parenteral and Enteral Nutrition identifies five responsibilities of the role of the NNS (Silk, 1994):

- Clinical practice
- Education
- Management (including audit)
- Acting as the patient's advocate
- Research

My role incorporates all these responsibilities, but some sections may fall into different categories, as discussed below.

Clinical practice

The basis of good clinical practice is to provide sound advice, written guidelines, policies and protocols which are research based and reviewed regularly to avoid them becoming out of date. For example, I have recently carried out an audit of the nursing care guidelines for the patient receiving a feed via a percutaneous endoscopic gastrostomy (PEG) as part of a larger audit (Arrowsmith & Tracey, 1997). This has identified a need for further study into the prevention of infection at the percutaneous endoscopic gastrostomy stoma site, which would include updating the nursing care guidelines.

Although my role is essentially hospital based I act as a specialist advisor on the nursing aspects of nutritional care in the community. If a patient is to be discharged on nutritional support (enteral or parenteral nutrition), I provide a training programme for the patient/carer and carry out a follow-up home visit when a patient is discharged to ensure that the patient/carer are coping and to provide training and support to the community nurses (nursing home or hospice staff if applicable). I also need to ensure the correct equipment is supplied to the patient in the community and that the funding for this is established. The discharge of the patient receiving enteral nutrition has been discussed elsewhere (Arrowsmith, 1994).

Another prime area of the role is to act as the patient's advocate and provide counselling and psychological support to the patient and/or carers when necessary in relation to their nutritional support. When a decision needs to be made as to whether a tube feed is going to benefit an elderly patient with an irreversible disease and a poor prognosis, the NNS can advise as part of the multi-disciplinary team and can also offer help and support to the family on this sensitive issue. The same dilemma can arise with regard to the provision of parenteral nutrition, for example in some critically ill patients or a patient with a non functioning gut approaching the terminal stages of AIDS. It is also necessary to help some patients decide which type of tube/line is most suitable for cosmetic reasons or ease of use, e.g. for a young adult patient with cystic fibrosis.

The NNS should have a sound knowledge of the feeding tubes and intravenous catheters available, and their insertion techniques, in order to advise the nursing and medical staff and/or patient of the most suitable device for their needs. For example, I recently organized an evaluation of a new nasogastric tube which was subsequently accepted for use in the hospital; however, I do assess its performance on an ongoing basis.

Up to now I have mainly discussed the role in an advisory capacity but most NNSs will have a clinical caseload which will incorporate advising and training staff and patients. I receive referrals directly via my pager, and these are initially seen within 24 hours and their subsequent care planned. I have here divided this area of the role into enteral and parenteral nutrition.

Enteral nutrition

If the patient is to receive or is already receiving an enteral tube feed they may be referred for the following reasons:

- To pass a nasogastric tube if intubation is difficult and has already been attempted by the ward nurse
- To replace or insert a gastrostomy feeding tube through an existing tract
- To review patients who have been referred for percutaneous endoscopic gastrostomy (PEG) to assess whether this is a suitable method of feeding for the patient and liaise with the referring team and family/carers as discussed above.

If a PEG is going to be placed, the patient and/or carers will be shown the gastrostomy, and its insertion and aftercare will be discussed. Several NNSs are involved in the PEG placement procedure itself by assisting with the procedure or inserting the gastrostomy tube under the endoscopist's guidance.

Parenteral nutrition

At Birmingham Heartlands Hospital the nutrition team (as mentioned above) carry out three ward rounds a week to receive referrals for parenteral nutrition, and subsequently monitor these patients. The team work together in decision-making, calculating nutritional requirements and formulation of the parenteral nutrition, i.e. ensuring correct fluid, electrolyte and trace element content. The team advises on intravenous access, suitable feeding catheters and monitoring, e.g. for signs of catheter infection, (intolerance to glucose), i.e. raised blood glucose – fluid and electrolyte imbalance and ability to tolerate enteral feeding.

My main responsibilities within the team are:

- Participation with the team in ensuring the patients who are referred are suitable for parenteral nutrition, and liaison with the referring team if an alternative route of feeding is suggested.
- Assessing venous access for a feeding catheter, considering the length of time parenteral nutrition will be required or assessing the suitability of an existing catheter (a previously used catheter may increase the risk of infection if parenteral nutrition is administered through it).
- Once a catheter has been chosen for placement I have been trained to insert some types of catheter, e.g. a peripheral midline (22 gauge, 20 cm long) catheter (Colagiovanni, 1996) or a peripherally inserted central catheter (Gabriel, 1996). A few NNSs are placing centrally placed tunnelled feeding catheters, e.g. Hamilton (1993).

There are two advantages of the nutrition nurse specialist placing the catheter: a reduction in catheter sepsis due to one expert practitioner performing the procedure, i.e. infection rates reduced to <1% (Hamilton, 1993); and increased quality of patient care. The process of catheter selection, informing/counselling the patient, placing the catheter and subsequent monitoring, nurse training on catheter care. The care of the patient receiving parenteral nutrition, are one complete episode of patient care managed by the nutrition nurse specialist.

Education

Education is incorporated into the clinical role of the NNS and involves the training of nurses, dietitians, doctors, other health care workers and patients and their carers. Formal classroom education reaches a larger audience, including nurses and health care workers from outside the Trust. I provide training sessions for trainee and qualified nurses in a variety of settings on English National Board courses, other post-registration courses and in-house training arranged at Birmingham Heartlands Hospital. The training usually covers all aspects of nutritional support from nursing assessment of nutritional status, i.e. the nutrition risk score used at Birmingham Heartlands Hospital (Reilly *et al.*, 1995) to the different routes used for nutritional support and the subsequent care of the patient receiving enteral or parenteral nutrition. I also organize training sessions in the ward areas if it is easier for the nurses; this enables all levels of nurses including health care assistants to attend.

At Birmingham Heartlands Hospital there are nutrition link nurses on each ward who are responsible for attending regular meetings to update them on current issues regarding nutritional support and thus act as a resource of information and expertise for their own ward area. I organize the meetings every three months and also encourage the nurses to spend some time working with me.

Research

As an expert in the field of nutritional support, the NNS should keep abreast of current issues and research projects carried out in this area. When developing and writing policies and protocols and prescribing patient care, where possible the NNS should carry out a thorough literature search on the relevant topic and base practice on relevant research findings. As a specialist practitioner NNSs are also in a position to facilitate and take part in research projects. Carrying out a literature search may help to identify problem areas that need further study to clarify the findings. Clinical audit can also identify areas that need further work, e.g. following the audit on infection at PEG stoma sites.

At Birmingham Heartlands Hospital I also audit every catheter used for parenteral nutrition for infection or other complications. Fortunately the infection and complication rate is low (2–6% per year) but if this were to change I would be looking for a reason why, which may require reviewing the literature and researching the use of different equipment, e.g. connections or catheter handling techniques.

Any areas of interest or study should be submitted for publication to a suitable nursing journal as this is another way of educating a wider audience and enhancing the practice of others. I have published several articles on nursing practice related to nutritional support, and the audit on PEG stoma site infection as an abstract.

Management

Time management and prioritizing workload are of prime importance whether the NNS is a lone practitioner or part of a nutrition team. Managing time can be difficult, particularly as patient referrals take priority, therefore planned work such as teaching may need to be rescheduled if there is no one else to deal with an urgent referral. Many NNSs, myself included, do not have secretarial support so this has to be fitted into my working day.

It is imperative that the NNS accurately documents any patient intervention in the medical and nursing notes, and if they keeps their own records, that patient confidentiality is maintained by safe storage. Patient records are essential for my yearly audit of the service, including patient outcomes. I produce a yearly report which is circulated to the relevant departments to update them, particularly on the service input to their own specialty. This has been useful in my recent bid to obtain funding for a second nutrition nurse due to increased patient referrals to the service.

Some NNSs may be budget holders for equipment and will need to ensure this is not overspent. In my area I have a limited budget whereby I keep specialist tubes and catheters and charge the ward/department when these are used in order to replenish my stock.

As well as the specific duties within this role the NNS, like any practising nurse, has accountabilities to the hospital trust which include adherence to the United Kingdom Central Council (UKCC) Code of Conduct, hospital policies and attending mandatory update sessions. NNSs has a further responsibility for their own professional development in relation to practice, e.g. attendance at relevant courses, study days and conferences. The need for the NNS to register as a specialist practitioner with the UKCC is currently an issue, as no special qualification exists. The benefits of degree level education cannot be emphasized enough in order to raise the profile of the NNS and give parity in working alongside other health care professionals. The national nurses nutrition group has been involved in the development of a BSc/MSc course in nutritional support which was launched in early 1998. The first students began the course in July 1998.

In conclusion, the role of the NNS within the multi-disciplinary team is essential to ensure that patients requiring nutritional support benefit from the NNS's expertise and receive a high standard of care.

References

Arrowsmith, H.L. (1994) Discharging patients receiving enteral nutrition. *British Journal of Nursing,* **3** (11), 551–7.

Arrowsmith, H. & Tracey, M. (1997) Percutaneous endoscopic gastrostomy (PEG) in

Birmingham Heartlands Hospital (BHH): assessment of the effectiveness and outcome of one dose of prophylactic antibiotics prescribed before PEG placement; evaluation of nursing care of stoma site and monitoring patient outcome. Abstract. *Proceedings of the Nutrition Society*, **56** (2).

Colagiovanni, L. (1996) Peripheral benefits. *Nursing Times*, **92** (4) (Nutrition Suppl. No. 2).

Gabriel, J. (1996) Care and management of peripherally inserted central catheters. *British Journal of Nursing*, **5** (10), 594–9.

Hamilton, H. (1993) Care improves while costs reduce; the clinical nurse specialist in total parenteral nutrition. *Professional Nurse*, June, 592–6.

Reilly, H.M., Martineau, J.K., Moran, A. & Kennedy, H. (1995) Nutritional screening – evaluation and implementation of a simple nutrition risk score. *Clinical Nutrition*, **14**, 269–73.

Silk, D.B.A. (Chairman and Editor) *Organisation of Nutritional Support in Hospital*. A report by a working party of the British Association for Parenteral and Enteral Nutrition, Maidenhead, Berks.

Chapter 13

Developing the Role of Lecturer Practitioner in Private Sector Health Care

Elizabeth Alsbury

Introduction

Nuffield Hospitals exist in a nationwide spread of 38 hospitals. A corporate body predetermines the general philosophy of providing a high standard of patient care at a reasonable cost. Each hospital is then autonomously managed by individual management teams, consisting of hospital manager, matron, business office manager, marketing manager and hotel services manager. Implementation of the underlying principles then becomes dependent on the strategies employed within each management structure.

Nursing principles within each hospital take into account individualized patient care, and nurses work generally with a case load of between four and six patients in any one shift. The main function of each hospital is acute surgery in a variety of disciplines. This means that in any shift nurses may be caring for the pre- and post-operative needs of patients undergoing general surgery, ophthalmics, ENT, gynaecology, orthopaedics, endoscopy and urology. Medical patients of all varieties are also admitted.

The fact that each patient is cared for by a consultant means that nurses and indeed the multi-disciplinary team are aware of two client groups – primarily the patients and secondarily the consultants – who also have individual requirements and needs. Most Nuffield Hospitals have 'inhouse' pharmacy, pathology, X-ray, health screening, outpatient facilities and physiotherapy, as well as hotel services. Clearly each has theatre suites and theatre sterilizing and supplies units. The multi-disciplinary teams work together in the same way as they do in NHS hospitals, although each unit is smaller and more compact.

Developing the role

With a background of stress management and counselling in addition to my role as theatre sister, I had developed a passion for education generally.

After 10 years in theatre, during which time I acquired my Certificate in Education, I assumed the role of lecturer-practitioner. During my theatre experience I also organized a considerable amount of education within the hospital for both ward and theatre staff.

The lecturer practitioner role enabled me to consolidate my educational learning and to liaise and network with other members of the multi disciplinary team, both within my own hospital and in other areas. In tandem with the new role I was also studying for my Masters Degree in Education in order to further qualify my educational commitment.

When I assumed the title lecturer practitioner, it was new to Nuffield Hospitals. I was given the autonomy and support required to evolve the role in a way which was appropriate to the requirements of the area in which I operated. Many areas needed attention and proactive support in the changing realms of health care. I was fascinated by the apparent need for theatre nurses to justify and expand their role, and the contrasting lack of motivation among them to do so. Geographical location and psychological barriers presented a huge challenge for theatre staff in integrating with the rest of the multi-disciplinary team of the hospital. The logistics of staffing levels and facilitating the often short-notice changes to theatre lists added to the apparent difficulties of integration.

The pre-admission clinic

Having regard for the challenges, I established a pre- and post-operative visiting service so that theatre staff had the opportunity to expand their role towards a more patient-centred approach. This provided the potential to liaise more closely with ward staff and other multi-disciplinary team players. In a short time, my idea expanded to the provision of a pre-admission clinic. The rationale for this was in providing a better timed facility, in which patients would benefit from physiological and psychological pre-assessment. Given time, patients would be more adequately informed and participate in their planned care throughout the whole operative event. Theatre staff, in liaison with ward staff, could use their special expertise in communicating with patients in the clinic setting. This included information about anaesthetists, operative procedures and recovery, including pain and symptom control in the immediate post-operative setting. Well timed assessment would also mean a reduction in potential case cancellation, due to physiological unsuitability of patients who would otherwise be admitted to hospital only a very short time before their planned operation.

Having communicated with consultants, theatre and ward staff, and the hospital matron, I found sufficient support for the idea to establish a pilot scheme for the clinic. The matron, out-patients manager, senior ward sister and myself met to establish protocols and principles for the clinic. Initially we invited patients in the 60+ age group to attend the clinic. Each patient was allocated an hour, during which a complete admission and assessment could be carried out. This meant that admission and discharge criteria were planned in discussion with the patient. A physical assessment was carried out, to include blood pressure, ECG, relevant history and appropriate blood tests. MRSA screening was completed if necessary, and all findings reported to relevant consultants.

My background in theatre meant that I could explain to patients relevant details regarding their operation, the procedures which would happen in the anaesthetic room and the immediate recovery period. I was able to discuss the use of intravenous infusion and oxygen in the recovery phase, and give clear guidelines related to pain control and symptom relief, as required by each individual. Patient information leaflets were also designed to reinforce this information. While ward or outpatient staff could complete the essential admission and discharge criteria, my theatre expertise enabled me to share with patients relevant details about the actual theatre experience.

The whole process was audited three months after the pilot scheme was launched. High satisfaction in all areas was revealed. Patients felt reassured and informed to the degree that they wished. The main anxieties experienced included pain and nausea control, the anaesthetic itself (many patients were concerned about waking during the procedure, or not waking up at all after the operation). Preparing patients in this sensitive but informed way appeared to lead to a smoother recovery and reduced pain and nausea.

Ward staff were delighted with a significant reduction in the 'hurry factor' when admitting these patients to hospital. The fact that all the paperwork and tests had been completed meant that the ward staff could build a better relationship of trust with their patients. Consultants revealed satisfaction with the risk assessment and advanced notice of deviations from 'normal' in blood pressure, ECG readings and blood screening. For theatre staff this was an opportunity to expand their role, to feel and become more involved with patients as individuals, and to become a more cohesive part of the whole team.

For my own professional development, the clinic was very progressive. My knowledge and skills increased in liaison with ward staff, physiotherapy and pathology. In tandem with the outpatients sister, I was soon able to fully participate in the whole admission procedure, including discharge criteria. Perceived difficulties in the logistics of theatre staffing and duty rostering resulted in my assuming a new role of ward sister. As such I was significantly empowered to participate in the clinic for two full days in each week. During this time I was able to give more energy to another development in establishing a pain/symptom control team within the hospital.

This resulted in a comprehensive pain control leaflet for patient information, and updating facilities for all staff in this important aspect of patient care.

My background in stress management and assertiveness training enabled me to assume a supportive and educational role as ward sister. Availability in an ordinary, everyday capacity resulted in ward staff asking the questions they had needed to address regarding theatre procedures. They reported satisfaction and empowerment from understanding why patients returned from theatre with pains and symptoms apparently unrelated to their procedures. Sore chins, aching legs and painful throats were among the apparently unrelated symptoms. I was also able to exchange knowledge related to actual operative procedures, and in exchange gained knowledge about post-operative recovery routines and length of patient stay.

Staff skills and empowerment

In the development of my counselling skills, I had followed the philosophy of Rogers (1982) whose work implied that, if individuals are given unconditional positive regard, they will be empowered to know how to solve their own life challenges. This underpinning personal philosophy enabled me to lead staff into self-empowerment, by encouraging them to realize their own worth, without unnecessary critical judgement of their ability or personality, but providing appropriate and relevant structure and help as and when required. These indirect elements of care in education, coupled with ongoing updating in whatever staff expressed a need for, have increased their knowledge and esteem. Resulting from this is improved patient care from a holistic baseline and increased medical confidence generally, which has been demonstrated in the establishment of a high dependency area and team. There is now a dedicated room with appropriate equipment, which is used on a regular basis. In order to facilitate this change, we have initially used the High Dependency Unit (HDU) area for ordinary major surgical cases. This has allowed staff to feel comfortable in the setting, with patients they would normally have nursed in an ordinary room. Confidence is increasing steadily.

Further improving the clinical skills of staff has included an in-house venepuncture course, which we plan to extend to cannulation. On top of the general updating and educational facilities, I periodically run staff support days centred on stress management and assertiveness. The stress management aspect of my work has most recently extended to establishing a stress management clinic. Patients are referred to this via their own GP or company occupational health schemes. Due to the profile of stress being raised among consultants, they are now requesting this as an in-patient service, which I facilitate when possible.

Conclusion

I feel sure that my profile as lecturer-practitioner, coupled with my commitment to education, has resulted in increased staff awareness and skill in these areas. For the future I would like to see the facilities extended to the development of a group of specialist nurses in areas such as breast care, stoma care, risk assessment, pain control and many others. These could be shared by our south-west division. In such a way I seek to advance the practice of nursing within Nuffield Hospitals. For my own development, as time allows, I would welcome the chance to become an advanced practitioner in risk assessment and pain control.

If I were to predict the future of the clinic, I would say that its expansion will continue. The clinic embraces three sessions per week, two of them whole days. Patients are invited from all age groups and surgical varieties, and all report high satisfaction levels. A mobile facility exists in which the full assessment is carried out with mobile equipment in the patient's own home. At the time of writing, the economic viability of this venture is being evaluated. Patient and consultant satisfaction are already concurrent with the continuation of this practice.

There are still many factors which need to be addressed in order to expand the role of the theatre nurse, and I will re-address those issues in the foreseeable future. There are equally many other issues to address, including the development of clinical supervision. The time, support and empowerment afforded by my own management team means that I shall continue to develop my role in relation to the required facilities within my own hospital, and perhaps within the south-west area as a whole. My life is constantly active and requires very careful time planning. It contains considerable variety and requires a good deal of stamina to keep pace with the clinical functions I must maintain, in tandem with the educational facility. The Nuffield Education Centre is in Wolverhampton and I visit frequently, which means a round trip of six hours in my car, and many more hours are spent visiting other hospitals. Despite this I remain motivated and enthusiastic within my ever changing and expanding role.

Reference

Rogers, C. (1982) *Freedom to Learn*. Charles E. Merrill, Columbus, Ohio.

Part 3
Advanced Practice

Always

Chapter 14
Advanced Practice in the UK

Paula McGee

Introduction

Advanced practice is defined by the UKCC as that in which the practitioner is engaged in:

'adjusting the boundaries for the development of future practice, pioneering and developing new roles responsive to changing needs and with advancing clinical practice, research and education, to enrich professional practice as a whole.' (UKCC, 1994)

Advanced practitioners are therefore seen by the Council as working at the frontline of the profession, trailblazing new elements of nursing and leading the way for others to follow. This requires considerable professional knowledge and expertise plus advanced education at master's level. Inevitably it is envisaged by the Council that only a small number of nurses will undertake this type of practice.

The concept of advanced practice is still quite new and there is debate about many issues in both British and American literature. The following five chapters, in Part 3, explore some of these through an examination of five examples of advanced practice as it is currently developing in the UK. It must be emphasized that each of the contributors presents only some aspects of her role and not a complete account of her work.

To begin with, the UKCC's definition implies a certainty about advanced practice which in reality does not exist. There is no standard, accepted definition of this form of nursing in North America where the term has been widely used for several years (Hamric, 1996), and within the UK, consensus about what the role should involve has yet to emerge (McGee *et al.*, 1996). Consequently the five nurses who present aspects of their roles in Part 3 reflect a diversity in development. What is certain is that some forms of nursing transcend specialization, even though they may be based in it. There is something beyond the possession of high levels of knowledge and expertise which enables the individual practitioner to function in a different way. The elusive nature of this difference has created difficulties in articulating its nature. Hamric (1996) proposes that, as with the nurse specialists, it is possible to identify a range of core elements within the advanced role. In her opinion 'advanced nursing practice is the application of an extended range of practical, theoretical and research based therapeutics to phenomena experienced by patients within a specialized clinical area of the larger discipline of nursing'.

Patricia Overton-Brown (Chapter 19) and Patricia Elliot (Chapter 18) share Hamric's view of a multi faceted advanced nursing role. Elliot sees advanced practice as an integration of practice, education, leadership, research and consultancy coupled with the individual practitioner's scope of practice and personal qualities. Patricia Overton-Brown sees it as holistic practice which incorporates education, research, consultancy and leadership. Advanced practice in her view is more than specialist nursing, which she sees as based on the medical model. Advanced practice is about what drives the individual, what motivates them. Thus for both these nurses advanced practice is not simply a set of skills and roles. It is 'a way of thinking and viewing the world based on clinical knowledge rather than a composition of roles' (Davies & Hughes, 1995) and demands an inquiring articulate mind with the ability to lead, show creativity, be flexible and take risks. Being an advanced practitioner is therefore as much about individual characteristics as professional expertise.

Expert coaching and guidance

The advanced practitioner has a broad teaching role which may incorporate both formal classroom work and interpersonal processes which may be summarized in the term 'coaching'. In particular, coaching is associated with helping nurses make transitions either from student to newly qualified staff nurse or from one set of working practices to another (Clarke & Spross, 1996). It is evident from the examples presented in Part 3 that all practitioners engage in formal classroom activity. Fiona Rich, as a lecturer (Chapter 17), obviously spends a considerable amount of time in teaching activities but there are other examples, such as Patricia Elliott's workshops on advanced health assessment skills (Chapter 18) and Patricia Overton-Brown's involvement in course development (Chapter 19).

The coaching function pervades all of these accounts with a strong emphasis on empowering staff. Kate Gee's coaching (Chapter 16) enables staff who do not work in coronary care, not simply to learn new skills required for thrombolysis but to incorporate them confidently into their practice. In a sense she preceptored the staff group, enabling them to contextualize new knowledge alongside their existing expertise (Benner *et al.*, 1996). To achieve this Kate Gee required high levels of competence in technical, clinical and interpersonal skills applied in a person-centred manner, which enabled her to transcend the differences between her and the staff (Clarke & Spross, 1996). It is this person-centredness which differentiates the coaching function in advanced practice from other types of teaching in displaying mastery of a complex web of knowledge and skills. Zukav (1979), in his book on quantum physics, says that a master/expert:

> 'is one who started before you did ... begins from the centre and not from the fringe. He imparts an understanding of the basic principles before going on ... in this way (he) dances with the student. (He) does not teach but the student learns.'

Clinical and professional leadership

The concept of empowering others to change their practice and act in the best interests of their patients is closely linked to leadership activities. Leadership requires:

- Vision (Malone, 1996), being able to see possibilities and opportunities in situations. Leaders present new ways of looking at everyday events and draw people's attention to new horizons. This may involve stepping over the traditionally accepted boundaries of nursing and forging new working alliances with members of other professional groups. Jenny La Fontaine's vision of the possibilities for elderly patients (Chapter 15) is a central element in bringing about changes in the way staff regard them. Sharing visions is an inspirational act through which the leader motivates others and persuades them to act.

- The use and employment of followers (Malone, 1996), which is axiomatic since leadership cannot be exercised without them. The advanced practitioner empowers others to achieve his or her vision and, in doing so, is challenged to present more details of it. Thus, as Jenny La Fontaine demonstrates (Chapter 15), working with followers allows them to gain in terms of personal and professional development but also to contribute meaningfully to the overall goal.

- The ability to take risks (Malone, 1996), which is important in situations where there is no blueprint for action. As Fiona Rich points out (Chapter 17), the advanced practitioner must be skilled at assessing the degree of risk involved and is responsible for selecting an appropriate course of action. Change cannot be achieved without some element of risk; a lack of risk might even be boring for some. The advanced practitioner may well enjoy the uncertainty that this aspect of the role brings but that enjoyment is modified by a knowledge of risk assessment and the application of research in developing standards, procedures and policies. The advanced practitioner can therefore modify courses of action to prevent or minimize harm.

- Mentoring less experienced staff by acting as a guide, coach, sponsor and advocate in both formal and informal settings (Malone, 1996). Patricia Elliot's work with the staff group (Chapter 18) could be regarded in this light as, through her leadership and coaching, they became empowered to interact more confidently with the medical staff. As a result, communication between doctors and nurses improved. Through her role as an advanced practitioner, Patricia Elliott had a vision of what could be achieved and was able to communicate that to the nurses. She was able to inspire them to try the advanced health assessment skills training, but was then sufficiently confident in her own ability to stand back and allow the nurses to practise what they had been taught. In doing so Patricia Elliott demonstrates an important principle in leadership – knowing when to take a back seat.

Consultation

The advanced practitioner is well placed to act as a resource, providing advice, guidance or education for patients, nurses and other health care professionals (Barron & White, 1996). This is possible because the advanced practitioner is not tied to the demands of a case load and can therefore adopt an indirect care role, influencing care through others, throughout the organization and at different levels (Koetters, 1989; McGee, 1995). In this context Fiona Rich's role (Chapter 17) has a strong element of indirect care and consultation since her work is mainly about empowering others. She has expertise which is recognized by others as valuable and has well-developed interpersonal skills which enable her to fulfil this aspect of her role. The responsibility she carries is enormous because the advice she gives must be accurate, appropriate, ethical, achievable and within the scope of practice.

Fiona Rich also highlights the frustrations of consultation in that she has no authority to direct and practitioners are free to choose other courses of action. Kate Gee (Chapter 16) also draws attention to this negative element in the consultation role. Her account shows that it is not enough to have the requisite knowledge and be recognized as an expert. She had to gain the respect of the staff in the admission unit. Introducing the new thrombolysis programme required managerial authority and Kate Gee's position in the nursing hierarchy helped her on both counts. As a senior nurse she had the power not only to advise but to implement courses of action.

The nature of advanced practice in the UK

It is evident from examining the five roles presented in Part 3 that some commonalities can be established with regard to coaching, consultation and leadership. It is also evident that there is considerable overlap between these elements. Empowerment of others, for example, is achieved through education but also through leadership. Consultation is closely linked with leadership in that both provide opportunities for the individual to influence others. Communication and interpersonal skills are central to the success of all three elements discussed and to advanced practice generally.

It is too early to say whether these five roles reflect developments in advanced practice throughout the UK. More research is needed to clarify this issue. Becoming an advanced practitioner could be seen as a development of the specialist nursing role. The nurse simply becomes more and more knowledgeable and adept at expert practice. Eventually the interface between nursing and medicine becomes blurred with significant overlaps in terms of decision-making, diagnostic and therapeutic skills, problem solving, research and education (Hunsberger *et al.*, 1992).

This view of advanced practice creates confusion between the two roles. A survey of NHS Trusts in England (McGee *et al.*, 1996) found that a number of respondents were concerned about lack of clarity between advanced and specialist roles which might lead to more fragmented care. The survey also showed that specialist nurses conformed to the sub-roles of care giver, teacher, researcher, consultant, leader and manager (Girard, 1987; Hamric & Spross, 1989), whereas the advanced role, in comparison, was not well defined and tended to be centred on medical tasks (McGee *et al.*, 1996). In addition, employing advanced practitioners, on senior grades, was seen as expensive and there seemed little incentive to fund posts which were not clearly differentiated from professional and specialist practice.

This is not solely a matter for the UKCC. Since the publication of the UKCC standards for post-registration, education and practice (UKCC, 1994), there has been an increasing number of posts entitled 'advanced practitioner'. In creating these posts, managers need to consider whether their expectations are truly in the realms of advanced practice, pioneering new aspects of nursing, or centred on replacing medical staff (McGee *et al.*, 1996).

It may be that making distinctions between specialist and advanced nursing is artificial, since both roles require the same level of expertise. The difference may be more a matter of emphasis within an individual role. For example, Watts *et al.* (1996) argue that the nurse specialist is 'nurse centred with emphasis on staff education, consultation, management and research'. In contrast the advanced practitioner has an expanded clinical role in 'advanced physical assessment, diagnosis and treatment' (Watts *et al.*, 1996) with less emphasis on other activities. In this context, specialist nurses and advanced practitioners are equal and, in some American states, legislation allows for this (Pearson, 1997). Each state has its own Nurse Practice Act and therefore developments are not standardized on a nationwide basis, but there does seem to be a trend to include clinical nurse specialists, advanced practitioners, nurse practitioners, nurse anaesthetists and nurse midwives under the title of advanced practitioner (Pearson, 1997). It is then possible to argue that specialist practice is not an essential stepping stone to advanced practice but a parallel career move.

Advanced practice must also be seen within the changing context of health care and in particular the need to reduce costs. The assumption here is that advanced practitioners can meet the 'everyday health care needs of people where they live and work' (Smith, 1995). In this context, advanced practitioners are first line providers of health services, able to assess, diagnose and treat a range of conditions. In North America advanced nurses in some states even have prescribing authority and are allowed to practice without direct medical supervision (Pearson, 1997).

Inevitably this raises the issue of the desirability of nurses taking on work normally done by doctors, and a host of unresolvable debates. What matters here is not professional protectionism but the circumstances in which work is passed from one staff group to another. Inherent in this must be consideration of:

- The maintenance of professionalism, safeguarding the welfare of the patient (Turnberg *et al.*, 1996).
- Clarity about the overlap of medical and nursing functions, health problems which do not require a doctor's intervention and what it is that both contribute to patient treatment and care (Pearson, 1995).
- The provision of education and training in that anyone taking on new roles/tasks must be properly trained to a nationally agreed standard (Turnberg *et al.*, 1996).
- Safety and standards in that there must be a system for monitoring performance on a regular basis (Turnberg *et al.*, 1996).
- Clarification of responsibility for actions (Turnberg *et al.*, 1996).
- A demonstration of the need for change (Turnberg *et al.*, 1996) and the ability to convince service purchasers that nurses are the most appropriate personnel to perform certain tasks. At the moment it is clear to purchasers what doctors do, but it is not clear what advanced practitioners do (Pearson, 1995).
- Clarification of the effectiveness of the changes and the costs involved (Turnberg *et al.*, 1996).
- Estimation of patient satisfaction with the changes and procedures which, where possible, should be compared with the level of satisfaction prior to the change (Turnberg *et al.*, 1996).

Issues for the future

Many factors will affect the successful development of the advanced practice role. PREP (UKCC, 1994) challenges nurses to clarify the overlap of roles between professional, specialist and advanced practice and state what is required from each type of practitioner (McGee, 1993). Different fields of practice will present diverse solutions to this challenge but nursing already has broad criteria for professional competence and Hamric's (1989, 1996) work suggests that this may be possible for specialist and advanced practice.

Developments in both nursing and medicine raise questions about the functions of both disciplines. What is it that we need a doctor for? Why do we need nurses? As both professions progress, it becomes more necessary to redefine those areas of health care which can be safely dealt with by a nurse and those which require medical intervention (Pearson, 1995). This clarification is essential as a prelude to intensive education of the public and the purchasers of health care, all of whom believe they understand what doctors do but who have little understanding of modern nursing capabilities (Pearson, 1995). If advanced practitioners are to be trusted by patients and accepted by purchasers, they must be able to demonstrate, in concrete terms, what they can provide.

Advanced practitioners will also need to develop professional groupings to promote their interests. At present the only general group which does this is the Specialist Nurses and Advanced Practitioners Association which seeks to unite advanced practitioners under a single umbrella. Such an approach is intended to foster and enhance the advanced practitioners' power base. This is in contrast to the North American situation where the creation of several advanced practice organizations has led to a fragmented situation (Pearson, 1995).

Conclusion

It is evident from this chapter that advanced practice is a complex activity incorporating several roles underpinned by a wide range of knowledge and skills. There is overlap between these roles, and attempting to separate them detracts from the holistic nature of advanced practice. Thus advanced practice is more than the sum of particular professional expertise and individual attributes, but more research is needed to explore it further.

References

Barron, A. & White, P. (1996) Consultation. In: *Advanced Nursing Practice. An Integrative Approach* (eds A. Hamric, J. Spross & C. Hanson) W.B. Saunders, Philadelphia.

Benner, P., Tanner, C. & Chesla, C. (1996) *Expertise in Nursing Practice. Caring, Clinical Judgement and Ethics.* Springer Publishing Company, New York.

Clarke, E. & Spross, J. (1996) Expert coaching and guidance. In: *Advanced Nursing Practice. An Integrative Approach* (eds A. Hamric, J. Spross & C. Hanson). W.B. Saunders, Philadelphia.

Davies, B. & Hughes, A. (1995) Clarification of advanced nursing practice: characteristics and competencies. *Clinical Nurse Specialist,* **9** (3), 156–60, 166.

Girard, N. (1987) The CNS: development of the role. In: *The Clinical Nurse Specialist: Perspectives on Practice* (ed. S. Menard). John Wiley and Sons, New York.

Hamric, A. (1996) A definition of advanced practice. In: *Advanced Nursing Practice. An Integrative Approach* (eds A. Hamric, J. Spross & C. Hanson). W.B. Saunders, Philadelphia.

Hamric, A. & Spross, J. (eds) (1989) *The Clinical Nurse Specialist in Theory and Practice,* 2nd edn. W.B. Saunders, Philadelphia.

Hunsberger, M., Mitchell, A., Blatz, S., Paes, B., Pinelli, J., Southwell, D., French, S. & Soluk, R. (1992) Definition of an advanced nursing practice role in the NICU: the clinical nurse specialist/neonatal practitioner. *Clinical Nurse Specialist,* **6** (2), 91–6.

Koetters, T. (1989) Clinical practice and direct patient care. In: *The Clinical Nurse Specialist in Theory and Practice,* 2nd edn (eds A. Hamric & J. Spross). W.B. Saunders, Philadelphia.

McGee, P. (1993) Defining nursing practice. *British Journal of Nursing,* **2** (20), 1022–3, 1026.

McGee, P. (1995) Are specialist nurses cost effective? Editorial. *British Journal of Specialist Nursing,* **4** (22), 1320.

McGee, P., Castledine, G. & Brown, R. (1996) *A survey of specialist and advanced nursing practice in England.* Report published by the Nursing Research Unit, University of Central England, Birmingham.

Malone, B. (1996) Clinical and professional leadership. In: *Advanced Nursing Practice. An Integrative Approach* (eds A. Hamric, J. Spross & C. Hanson). W.B. Saunders, Philadelphia.

Pearson, L. (1995) Annual update of how each state stands on legislative issues affecting advanced nursing practice. *Nurse Practitioner,* **20** (1).

Pearson, L. (1997) Annual update of how each state stands on legislative issues affecting advanced nursing practice. *Nurse Practitioner,* **22** (1).

Smith, M. (1995) The core of advanced nursing practice. *Nursing Science Quarterly,* **8** (1), 2–3.

Turnberg, L., Evans, J., Cameron, I., Ward, J., Hancock, C. & Winder, E. (1996) Skillsharing. Joint statement from the Royal College of Physicians London and the Royal College of Nursing. *Journal of the Royal College of Physicians of London,* **30** (1), 57.

UKCC (1994) *The Future of Professional Practice – the Council's Standards for Education and Practice Following Registration.* United Kingdom Central Council for Nursing, Midwifery and Health Visiting, London.

Watts, R., Hanson, M., Gallagher, S. & Foster, D. (1996) The critical care nurse practitioner: an advanced role for the critical care nurse. *Dimensions of Critical Care Nursing,* **15** (1), 48–56.

Zukav, G. (1979) *The Dancing Wu Li Masters.* Rider and Co., London.

Chapter 15

Advanced Practice in Working with Older People with Dementia

Jenny La Fontaine

Introduction

In working with older people with dementia, it can be argued that nurses experience the 'triple jeopardy' that Norman (1985) refers to when describing the experience of ageing. By this I mean that there are three constructs which have combined to create a blinkered and frequently negative attitude towards nursing this client group: ageism, psychiatry and traditional nursing.

Ageism

Research has demonstrated that ageism is a major part of the experience of ageing for older people in the UK (Bytheway, 1995). This research has also shown that ageism is inherent within health care in many areas of practice (Bytheway, 1995). This has manifested itself in various ways, for example refusing an older person certain types of treatment, but is particularly prevalent in the covertly and sometimes overtly expressed views and actions of the professionals who do not work with older people, and about their colleagues who practise in this area. Frequently nurses who work with older people are seen as unskilled and incapable of working in the more 'demanding' areas of nursing.

Perhaps the most obvious example of how nurses are affected by ageism is in that of resourcing. It is well recognized that older people rarely get the resources that would enable staff to offer the support they are entitled to (Bytheway, 1995). Frequently areas of care for older people have high ratios of unqualified to qualified staff which, while created by poor resourcing, serves to reinforce the view that care for older people is mainly unskilled work.

Psychiatry

The discrimination referred to in relation to ageism is also prevalent in psychiatry. Again, it is evident that mental illness carries a stigma (Birchwood & Tarrier, 1994), and has done so for many hundreds of years. The documented accounts of the way in which people with mental illness have been treated, both in the past and more recently, are a stark reminder of this. This discrimination has also had its impact on the staff who work with these people, who are often viewed as second class nurses.

Traditional nursing

As in many other areas, nursing in old age psychiatry has been dominated by the medical model. While this model has been of some use in addressing symptomatic aspects of the disorder, it has served to create a reductionist approach to the care of older people with dementia. Within this framework, dementia is seen as a disease that will cause an inevitable and irreparable decline in cognition and personality, and that is impervious to any actions that we as professionals may take. Within this framework, the response of nursing has been that of a custodial one, where efforts have been directed at protectionism and a focus on lost skills and abilities. Efforts to change this have met with difficulties. The introduction of reality orientation (RO) in the early 1980s was welcomed as a new and exciting approach to working with older people with dementia. However, with nurses still ingrained in the medical model approach, RO became yet another way of highlighting the individuals' deficits and of viewing what staff do as having little or no impact on the experience of dementia for the older persons in their care.

Impact and implications

I would suggest, therefore, that these three constructs have combined to make it unlikely that nursing older people with dementia could have been seen as an area in which advanced practice could occur. However, over the past 10 years changes have occurred. Psychiatry has in general moved towards a psychosocial model of care. This has been taken even further in working with older people with dementia by Kitwood & Bredin (1992). They have developed a theory of dementia care in which the central construct is that of personhood. They argue that older people with dementia are individuals first and foremost, and that they have the ability to experience a sense of personhood and therefore wellbeing, even into the later stages of dementia. They further suggest in their theory that the actions of the persons who care for these people can either enhance this sense of personhood or indeed can detract from it through their communication with that person.

This theory has at its core one of the fundamental skills of nursing, that of the ability to communicate with clients in order to develop a therapeutic relationship and therefore enable their needs to be met. Yet consistently research has shown that nurses communicate less, and the quality of those interactions declines when the person they are caring for is cognitively impaired (Jones, 1992).

As a lecturer in nursing and as a practitioner, this posed important questions for me and for the staff that I worked with and taught:

(1) Why do nurses find it difficult to communicate with older people who are severely impaired?
(2) Is communicating with older people who have dementia an inherent skill, or is it a developed skill which requires a conscious, intentional, reflective and creative approach that, at its most effective, is characteristic of advanced nursing practice?

The first question has in part been answered by Kitwood & Bredin (1992) in their discussion of their theory. They argue that staff bring their own set of problems to the scenario, i.e. their own baggage. This baggage frequently includes a fear of ageing, of death and of dementia, along with our own personal histories, all of which affect our ability to communicate openly with an individual. It is further suggested that communication implies a two-way exchange and that we place a high emphasis on our ability to communicate verbally. Where clients are unable to respond in this way, due to cognitive or other deficits, the reinforcers that would continue the exchange are not present. Even though we might recognize these difficulties, we have not necessarily developed the skills to alter our response in order to maintain the communication.

Kitwood argues that in order to be able to respond openly, staff need to develop a conscious awareness of their own difficulties that they bring to the situation, in much the same way that psychotherapists are required to do in order to practise effectively.

The second question above has been answered by other researchers, notably Jones (1992) and Savage (1995), who describe the fundamental importance of communication and the extent to which this can be creatively used to enhance the relationship between the client and the member of staff. Savage (1995) describes the conscious and intentional use of the variety of different ways that we can offer communication and listening, that goes beyond simple verbal communication, as something that is a developed skill. Jones (1992) discusses the extent to which nurses are frequently unable to communicate with people who have, among other difficulties, moderate to severe dementia, and presents a model of communication which is designed to overcome these difficulties.

Having had the opportunity to observe nursing staff interacting with people with dementia, both through the use of dementia care mapping (Kitwood & Bredin, 1992) and in discussions with nursing staff about how they developed their communication with clients, I found much informal evidence to support the research findings. The issues raised for me concerns about how I should utilize this knowledge to improve the care of clients with dementia.

Relevance to practice

The University of Birmingham (1996) master's in health sciences programme, which leads to the recognition of course participants as advanced practitioners, identifies in its continuous practice assessment that the characteristic that defines an advanced practitioner is that of innovation:

> 'The student demonstrates evidence of advanced nursing practice through pioneering and developing new roles responsive to changing needs.' (adapted from Steinaker & Bell, 1979)

I identified three areas in which this knowledge could be utilized to develop the skills of nurses, including myself, in order to enable staff to consciously and creatively communicate with clients, as described here.

Reflective practice

The use of reflective practice is an inherent part of self development. If I was to teach others about communication with people with dementia, it was important that I continued to analyse my own practice, and that I did this during my interactions with clients, to ensure that I was using appropriate responses. Two examples, which I subsequently used as critical incidents, served to highlight specific issues that I raised earlier, in relation to clients whose ability to verbally communicate was compromised because of their cognitive impairment.

First, a lady who had been an inpatient for a number of years and was considered to be very difficult to nurse. She frequently called out for a nurse and when one answered, she would verbally and physically abuse them. She also tended to shout out 'I'm bad' at the top of her voice. Her behaviour led to nurses avoiding contact unless necessary. I was carrying out dementia care mapping (Kitwood & Bredin, 1992) and was observing her. It was very clear that she desired some form of contact, but her verbal skills were impoverished. I sat next to her and touched her arm. I called her by name and asked if she felt bad. She pushed my hand away and said no. I then asked if she thought she was bad and she said yes. I asked why, and she said she missed her husband. She then cried, and allowed me to touch her and stroke her back. The member of staff who observed this said that she had never mentioned her husband before and had not allowed anyone to respond to her in that way. For some time after that she was calmer, shouted less and was active in seeking eye contact with others.

Secondly, a gentleman, who had also been an inpatient for some time, had lost the ability to verbally communicate and also had great difficulty in having contact with staff, particularly female staff. He was also one of the clients I observed in the process of dementia care mapping. He appeared throughout the time I was observing him to be watching me. After some time, I went and sat next to him and handed him the paper I was writing on and a pen. He took these and spent some time drawing. He drew nothing that was recognizable, but he interacted in a way that he had probably not had the opportunity to do before.

What was important about both of these incidents was not that they were particularly out of the ordinary in terms of the interaction, but that they highlighted that, through the conscious consideration of the client, communication can take place, even with people who are severely impaired, and that the outcome for these clients was an opportunity to express themselves and hopefully to experience wellbeing. In addition, it highlighted that if we expect to be able to achieve the same standard of communication that we have with our peers, then we are setting up both the client and ourselves for failure. We need to change the emphasis of our expectations and be creative in how we communicate. This allows us the opportunity to view each and every attempt that the client makes as an opportunity to communicate and experience an exchange. I continue to utilize reflection in my practice with people with dementia as a way of evaluating the responses that I make to clients so that I am as flexible and as creative as possible.

Developing communication skills

The use of dementia care mapping highlighted that communication was an area that staff needed to develop in order to respond to clients' needs more effectively. While many staff on the unit where this took place had previously attended courses in which communication skills were a component, it was clear that this did not always allow them the opportunity to implement what was learned or to develop their skills in a co-ordinated way. I therefore developed a training course in consultation with staff, which involved theoretical components but was primarily experiential based. It required staff to utilize critical incidents from their own experience. All the nurses on the unit attended the sessions, and as part of their commitment to their own development agreed to attend meetings which involved discussion of critical incidents from their own practice. During these meetings, analysis of those incidents and suggestions for practice were discussed. The workshops had the advantage of being solely focused on this client group, and were evaluated by staff as very positive and beneficial.

The next stage of the objective was to repeat the use of dementia care mapping to see if the experience of care had improved as a direct consequence of this and other achievements.

Influencing student nurses' experiences

Finally, a part of my role as a lecturer-practitioner involved the management of the education-led practice component of the Registered Mental Nurse Diploma. I was concerned that many students had a very negative view of working with older people, and viewed their placement with some trepidation. Many students expressed the view that they did not know what to say or how to communicate. In conjunction with a staff nurse on the unit, I developed an experiential based component of the module for older people, that involved almost 2 days of training on communication with older people and communication skills (out of a 10 day module) and further follow-up of analysis of their communication skills with their assessors and myself on a regular basis during their placement.

Conclusion

In conclusion, it is my view that working with older people with dementia, far from being an area which requires no skills, is in fact one which requires the development of a fundamental skill in nursing, that of communication. This skill is one that is rarely learned by the time a nurse has finished training, and indeed it could be argued that it is only at this point that it actually begins to develop in a coherent way. In order for nurses to develop advanced practice with older people who suffer with dementia, they need to focus on the following points:

(1) Their attitudes and values towards their own ageing and older people in order to recognize their own inherent ageism
(2) The use of reflective practice in such forums as clinical supervision
(3) The development of the conscious and intentional use of the skills of communication that go beyond that of verbal communication, in order to truly listen and hear what is being expressed

References

Bytheway, B. (1995) *Ageism*. Open University Press, Buckingham.
Birchwood, M. & Tarrier, N. (1994) Making a reality of the community management of schizophrenia. In: *Psychological Management of Schizophrenia* (eds M. Birchwood & N. Tarrier). Wiley Press, Sussex.
Jones, G. (1992) A communication model for dementia. In: *Caregiving in Dementia, Research and Applications* (eds G. Jones & B.M.L. Miesen). Routledge, London.

Kitwood, T. & Bredin, K. (1992) Towards a theory of dementia care, personhood and wellbeing. *Ageing and Society,* **12**, 269–87.

Norman, A. (1985) *Triple Jeopardy, Growing Old in a Second Homeland.* Centre for Policy on Ageing, London.

Savage, J. (1995) *Nursing Intimacy, an Ethnographic Approach to Nurse Patient Interaction.* Scutari Press, London.

Steinaker, N.W. & Bell, M.R. (1979) *The Experiential Taxonomy; a new approach to teaching and learning.* Academic Press, New York.

University of Birmingham (1996) *Post Experience Diploma in Health Sciences/Masters in Health Sciences (Advanced Practices) Guidelines for Pathway Supervisors.* Department of Nursing, Unpublished Paper, School of Health Sciences, University of Birmingham.

Chapter 16

The Roles of Consultant and Researcher in Advanced Practice Cardiology Nursing

Kate Gee

One of the challenges facing the advanced nurse practitioner is ensuring that their profession, organization and the patients they serve can evaluate their role. Research can provide a vehicle for such evaluation, although Wilson-Barnett *et al.* (1990) argue that for research findings to have a real impact on care, researchers need to face the realities of practice and service. Successful research in practice requires addressing issues that are based on practical, clinical problems, and that reflect what nurses want, need or value (Wilson-Barnett *et al.* 1990). However, researching such issues is unlikely to produce the precise definitions or accurate measurements which the United Kingdom Central Council (UKCC, 1996) recommends as requirements when evaluating the advanced nursing practitioner (ANP). Such evaluations are founded in positivist research methodologies that have gained success and recognition within health care (Buchanan, 1992).

This chapter will discuss my role as an advanced nurse practitioner in cardiology, from the perspectives of consultant and researcher. The context of this discussion will be the change in nursing practice within the clinical reality of care required by patients admitted to hospital experiencing an acute myocardial infarction who need thrombolysis. The practice change is related to the transference of responsibility for care of these patients from the specialist nursing staff in the coronary care unit to the generalist nurses working in the admission areas. The terms 'specialist' and 'generalist' in this context relate to the nature of nursing in each area rather than to specific qualifications (UKCC, 1996).

Thrombolytic therapy has revolutionized the clinical management of patients suffering from acute myocardial infarction. The restoration of coronary circulation achieved by prompt thrombolysis because of destruction of the coronary artery thrombus has dramatically reduced the incidence of death and complications associated with acute myocardial infarction (Snyder *et al.*, 1995; Simmons *et al.*, 1995; de Bono & de Bono,

1988). The dramatic reductions in mortality and morbidity associated with thrombolysis have reinforced the need to minimize the delay in commencing thrombolysis in suitable patients on their arrival at hospital. Since clinical management of acute myocardial infarction patients with complications is associated with technologically complex and therefore more expensive interventions (Meheswaran *et al.*, 1995; Pickin & St Leger, 1993; Wittels *et al.*, 1990), prompt thrombolysis not only improves patient recovery but reduces costs (Meheswaran *et al.*, 1995; GUSTO Investigators, 1993). Clinical audit of thrombolysis has also evolved because effective thrombolysis provides more effective and economical care (Meheswaran *et al.*, 1995).

Within the context of my ANP role I had responsibility for auditing thrombolysis. The audit tool was designed using the Donabedian (1980) framework. The audit focused on examining the diagnostic 'process' leading to thrombolysis so that reasons for delay were identified. This process depended on prompt electrocardiograph recording, referral to medical staff and effective clinical decision-making. In 1995, audit results suggested that delay occurred because thrombolysis was being started after the patient had been transferred to the coronary care unit from the admission area. Medical staff therefore decided to commence thrombolysis in the two admission areas, which were either the acute medical admissions unit or the accident and emergency department.

The success of this change required admission nurses to accept responsibility for patient supervision that had previously been undertaken by coronary care unit nurses. The clinical directors asked me to lead and evaluate this initiative through the audit process I had developed. Transference of responsibility required admission nurses to develop the psychomotor and assessment skills necessary to promote appropriate patient selection, prepare the infusion, and detect and manage complications associated with thrombolysis. Implementation and evaluation of this practice change will be discussed within the context of my consultant and researcher roles as the cardiology ANP.

The UKCC (1996) suggests that the consultant role of the advanced nurse practitioner is fundamental to advancing practice focused on boundary adjustments between professional groups in response to technological/scientific innovations. However, in this change scenario, my consultant and researcher roles were used to explore the transference of responsibility for acute myocardial infarction patients within the same professional group of nurses, who were working in different clinical areas. Walsh (1994) defines consultation as 'a process of communication between professionals'.

Three factors described by Egan *et al.* (1981), and cited by Wabscall (1987), as 'organizational conditions', legitimized my role as consultant within the organization:

(1) As a cardiac specialist nurse I was recognized as an expert in patient management following acute myocardial infarction
(2) As the leader of the thrombolysis audit I was already recognized within the multi-disciplinary team and understood the processes involved
(3) As a clinician on the coronary care unit I was in an ideal position to access the patient group, as they would be transferred from admission areas to the coronary care unit.

Although my credibility and legitimacy to lead this change were established within the organization (Sommer, 1983), I had to gain legitimacy with the admission nurses themselves. Since I was unable to work clinically with them, it was essential to select a research methodology that would enable me to gain meaningful insight into the contextual nature of their practice. The research methodology had to enable me to consider the situation from the admission nurses' perspective and value systems (Waterman, 1995; Dey, 1993), and also minimize any biases I may have had because of my coronary care unit background (Reardon, 1991), because:

> '... you never really know a man until you stand in his shoes and walk around in them.' (Lee, 1974)

Application of both qualitative and quantitative methods was required to collect evidence that could not only predict outcomes (UKCC, 1996), but also provide information that could contribute to the body of knowledge related to the transference of nursing responsibility from a specialist to generalist group of nurses (Buchanan, 1992). The research approach I selected was 'action research' as it promoted active participation of admission nurses (Hart & Bond, 1995). Involvement of admission nurses would enable them to make discriminating decisions regarding how they wanted their practice to respond when caring for patients requiring thrombolysis. This would minimize the risk of viewing the practice development as 'task' acquisition (Trofino, 1993; UKCC, 1992; Wilson-Barnett *et al.*, 1990).

Participation was particularly important as admission nurses had not been actively involved in the decision to commence thrombolysis in their areas. However, it would be unreasonable to criticize the actions of medical staff as they were also under pressure, not only to maximize therapeutic benefit but also to change practice to comply with purchaser demands, an economical pressure recognized as a potent influence on change (Handy, 1990). The intrusion of the forces of supply and demand imposed their own influences on the scope of both medical and nursing practice (Wainwright, 1994).

Since the success of medical practice depended on admission nurses accepting responsibility for patients requiring thrombolysis, admission nurse involvement was essential as lack of consultation can inhibit change (Bowman, 1995). For as Handy (1990) states:

'It is tempting to impose our goals on other people, particularly if they are subordinates ... the strategy will however be self defeating ... they may have to comply but they will not change.' (p. 59)

The participatory nature of action research made it possible to establish an active support system in which I was able to identify and act on admission nurses' ideas and concerns (Fenton, 1985). As action research advocated the application of several methods, i.e. triangulation, to promote positive change within a dynamic setting, I was able to explore the impact of this transference of nursing responsibility from various perspectives (Morse, 1994). To gain contextual meaning I designed and implemented an anonymous questionnaire, which enabled exploration of admission nurse attitudes towards thrombolysis being commenced in their area. Respondents also had the opportunity to make written comments about their feelings towards the attitude statements contained in the questionnaire, and could also select and prioritize teaching strategies which they felt could be used to meet *their* learning needs related to caring for patients requiring thrombolysis.

Comments mobilized by the attitude statements in the questionnaire suggested that admission nurses considered provision of resources, including suitably qualified, competent nurses to care for patients, important within their changeable working environment, where medical staff attendance was not guaranteed because of their workload. In general, admission nurses considered the coronary care unit environment and coronary care unit nurses as being more appropriate to supervise patients, and were opposed to taking responsibility for patients requiring thrombolysis, without additional training and resources. A thrombolysis workshop was designed that focused on addressing the issues and learning needs identified by the admission nurses in the questionnaire.

Five thrombolysis workshops were undertaken over five months, and 39 of 79 admission nurses attended. Workshop evaluation involved nurses making written comments on how they thought attending the workshop would impact on their practice. Thrombolysis audit was used as an independent variable to measure whether workshop intervention had improved organizational performance (Wood & Brink, 1989). Workshop impact comments suggested admission nurses had experienced increased perceptions of confidence, awareness, knowledge base and appreciation of the benefits of thrombolysis, with a decrease in perceptions of fear and panic in two instances.

The comments inferred that the teaching strategies I had used had enhanced perceptions of confidence towards electrocardiograph interpretation, and assertion skills with regard to interaction with medical staff.

These comments suggested admission nurses were more likely to refer patients to medical staff because of their improved electrocardiograph interpretation skills, and that they felt more able to detect side effects and identify contraindications. Within the context of Benner (1984), these inferences suggested practice enhancement was likely within the domains of the diagnostic monitoring function, administering and monitoring therapeutic regimen and the helping role. In some instances admission nurses made explicit statements regarding their abilities to interpret electrocadiographs, and question medical staff.

Audit analysis established that during the workshop intervention period (September 1995 to January 1996) delays between patient admission and electrocardiograph recording were reduced by 5%, and electrocardiograph recording to medical assessment improved by 9% within the first 30 minutes of arrival. These improvements suggested that the inferred behavioural changes indicated in the post-workshop comments had been implemented in practice. Most importantly, following workshop intervention there was an overall improvement of 19% in admission to thrombolysis at 30 minutes.

Action research allowed me to use my advanced coronary care unit skills to promote admission nurse practice. As a consultant my role embraced what Caplan (1970) describes as 'consultee-centred administrative' skills in that I was able to use my skills to guide and support admission nurses. This included providing advice regarding the type of infusion pumps to purchase, and assisting in the design of a multi-disciplinary therapeutic protocol and audit tool modification. My consultative role appeared to promote effective inter-departmental communication networks.

As an advanced nurse practitioner acting as a consultant and researcher, my involvement appeared to lead to improvements in organizational performance, and increased admission nurses' perceptions of confidence, competence and knowledge. Admission nurses were able to advance their practice because of a positive, proactive approach that recognized their contribution to care. Action research enabled me to apply my expertise to empower admission nurses to determine their own way forward, which Morse (1994) would describe as 'process consultation'. As Buchanan (1992) states:

> 'It is more demanding to ask people to grapple with uncertain judgements about whether a particular interpretation does justice to the complexity of human interaction.' (p. 133)

Action research promoted what Kincheloe and McLaren (1994) describe as 'critical trustworthiness', as interpretative analysis of admission nurse comments provided credible portrayals of the clinical realities facing the admission nurse. Collective consciousness of admission nurses appeared raised in relation to the importance of thrombolysis and their crucial role as the patients' advocate by encouraging their active participation in the change process. Over the five-month period of workshop intervention, the percentage of thrombolysis commenced in admission areas increased by 49%.

Although focused on a small modification in practice, within one Trust, my role as researcher and consultant highlighted important issues regarding the practice change scenario and the role of the nurse. Nurses face increasing pressure to change practice in relation to the introduction of technological and medical advancements in health care organizations, and thrombolysis represents only one such advance. By using an appropriate research methodology and process consultation I was able, as the advanced nurse practitioner in cardiology, to advance the practice of nurses working in a different clinical area. Practice advancement was achieved by having mutual professional respect, not only for admission nurses but for all the disciplines involved in thrombolysis, and by recognizing and utilizing their unique contribution to improving patient care delivery. Such an approach requires commitment and investment in staff through the application of a collaborative educative framework.

References

Benner, P. (1984) *From Novice to Expert: Excellence and Power in Clinical Nursing Practice.* Addison-Wesley, Menlo Park.

Bowman, M. (1995) *The Professional Nurse, Coping with Change, Now and in the Future.* Chapman & Hall, London.

Buchanan, D.R. (1992) An uneasy alliance: combining qualitative and quantitative research methods. *Health Education Quarterly,* **19** (1), 117–35.

Caplan, G. (1970) *The Theory and Practice of Mental Health Consultation.* Basic Books, New York.

de Bono, D. (1990) *Practical Thrombolysis.* Blackwell Science, Oxford.

de Bono, D. & de Bono, A. (1988) Coronary thrombosis. *The Practitioner,* **232**, 1099–1101.

Dey, I. (1993) *Qualitative Data Analysis.* Routledge, London.

Dimond, B. (1990) *Legal Aspects of Nursing.* Prentice Hall, Hemel Hempstead.

Donabedian, A. (1980) *Explorations in quality assessment and monitoring.* Health Administration Press, Michigan.

Egan, E.C., McElmurry, B.J. & Jameson, H.M. (1981) Practice-based research: assessing your department's readiness. *Journal of Nursing Administration,* **11** (10), 26–36.

Fenton, M.V. (1985) Identifying competencies of clinical nurse specialists. *Journal of Nursing Administration,* **15** (12), 31–7.

GUSTO Investigators (1993) An international randomised trial comparing four thrombolytic strategies for acute myocardial infarction. *New England Journal of Medicine,* **329** (10), 673–82.

Handy, C. (1990) *The Age of Unreason.* Arrow Books, London.

Hart, E. & Bond, M. (1995) *Action Research for Health and Social Care.* Open University Press, Buckingham.

Kincheloe, J.L. & McLaren, P.L. (1994) Rethinking critical theory and qualitative research. In: *Handbook of Qualitative Research* (eds N.K. Denzin & Y.S. Lincoln). Sage Publications, Newbury Park.

Lee, H. (1974) *To Kill a Mocking Bird.* Pan Books, UK.

Meheswaran, S., Chambers, J. & Weil, J. (1995) Getting there on time – reducing 'pain to door' delay. *British Journal of Health Care Management,* **1** (8), 392–4.

Morse, J.M. (1994) Designing funded qualitative research. In: *Handbook of Qualitative Research* (eds N.K. Denzin & Y.S. Lincoln). Sage Publications, Newbury Park.

Pickin, C. & St Leger, S. (1993) *Assessing Health Needs Using the Life Cycle Framework.* Open University Press, Buckingham.

Reardon, K.K. (1991) *Persuasion in Practice.* Sage Publications, Newbury Park.

Simmons, J., Willens, H.J. & Kesler, K.M. (1995) Acute myocardial infarction; then and now. *Chest,* **107** (6), 1732–43.

Snyder, M.L. & Hargrove Deelstra, M. (1995) Interventional cardiology techniques. In: *Cardiac Nursing,* 3rd edn (eds S.L. Woods, S. Froelicher, C.J. Halpenny, U. Motzer). Lippincott, Philadelphia.

Sommer, R. (1983) Action research is formative: research at the Saskatchewan Hospital, 1957–61. *Journal of Applied Behavioural Science,* **19** (4), 427–38.

Trofino, J. (1993) Transformational leadership: the catalyst for successful change. *International Nurse Review,* **40** (6), 179–87.

UKCC (1992) *The Scope of Professional Practice.* UKCC, London.

UKCC (1996) *The Nature of Advanced Practice, an Interim Report.* UKCC, London.

Wabscall, J.M. (1987) The CNS as researcher. In: *The Clinical Nurse Specialist, Perspectives in Practice* (ed. S.W. Menard). Chapman and Hall, New York.

Wainwright, P. (1994) Professionalism and the concept of role extension. In: *Expanding the Role of the Nurses* (eds G. Hunt & P.Wainwright). Blackwell Science, Oxford.

Walsh, S.M. (1994) The critical care clinical specialist role in consultation. In: *The Clinical Nurse Specialist Role in Critical Care* (eds A. Gawlinski & L.S. Kern). W.B. Saunders, Philadelphia.

Waterman, H. (1995) Distinguishing between 'traditional' and action research. *Nurse Researcher Compendium,* **2,** 97–205.

Wilson-Barnett, J., Corner, J. & DeCarle, B. (1990) Integrating nursing research and practice – the role of the researcher as teacher. *Journal of Advanced Nursing,* **15,** 621–5.

Wittels, E.H., Hay, J.W. & Gotto, A.M. (1990) Medical costs of coronary artery disease in the United States. *American Journal of Cardiology,* **65** (7), 432–40.

Wood, M.J. & Brink, P.J. (1989) Comparative designs. In: *Advanced Design in Nursing Research* (eds P.J. Brink & M.J. Wood). Sage Publications, Newbury Park.

Chapter 17

The Role of Advanced Nurse Practitioners in Learning Disability Nursing

Fiona Rich

The role of the advanced nurse practitioner in the field of learning disabilities is not necessarily that of a direct carer. However, as an advanced nurse practitioner it is possible to influence the care of people with learning disabilities through the use of empowerment and education.

An important distinction between the role of the registered nurse (mental handicap) (RNMH) and that of the advanced nurse practitioner is the possession of power, authority and autonomy to act in the greatest interests of clients and staff, together with a willingness to stand accountable for decisions made. Often nursing staff are faced with dilemmas of competing professional loyalties because of the power influences that inhibit individuals in the profession, i.e. management hierarchy, the medical profession and the restrictions that the nursing profession imposes on nurses in the form of codes of conduct, nursing policies and procedures (Miller *et al.*, 1983). As a result of these power influences, nursing staff all too often deny clients their rights because they feel powerless to take risks and advocate for the clients against policies, procedures or management hierarchy.

An advanced nurse practitioner can use his or her power, authority and autonomy to *indirectly* empower the RNMH to act in the greatest interests of clients and take controlled and calculated risks. This empowerment is achieved through being present in the clinical area and involves supporting staff in clinical decision-making through linking practice and education, i.e. by identifying, applying and disseminating research findings relating to clinical practice.

The necessity to maintain an indirect role in empowering the RNMH results from the perceived gap between the RNMH and the advanced nurse practitioner. This perceived gap is even more pronounced if the advanced nurse practitioner has a dual lecturer-practitioner role with another organization, as the advanced nurse practitioner will seem very distant to the RNMH. The gap is often perceived to be so great that there is a need for a further layer of professional practice which retains authority, i.e. the specialist nurse practitioner. The specialist nurse practitioner holds the delegated power and authority to act and intervene on behalf of clients and staff. The advanced nurse practitioner on the other hand is not necessarily in the position to act as a risk-taker directly, but influences policy and decision-making sufficiently to empower those who are directly involved in the process of risk-taking and to act decisively in morally difficult decisions. The reader should refer to Table 17.1 throughout the remainder of this chapter.

Looking at outcome 5 of the UKCC's (1994) standards for advanced nurse practitioners, there is a requirement to:

'supervise the clinical practice of the team to ensure safety and effectiveness in care and to identify individual and team development needs.'

This obligation cannot be fulfilled without the ability to empower staff to act in the best interests of clients. Empowerment requires staff to feel committed to philosophies of care, policies and procedures of service provision. As an advanced nurse practitioner, it is necessary to ensure that staff are involved in the development of services, policies and philosophies of care in order to establish the commitment of staff. From the advanced nurse practitioner point of view, this involves leading a small co-opted team of clinicians and managers who promote policy development and monitoring with the service managers and care staff.

Ensuring safety and effectiveness in care, however, implies a degree of risk-taking which is a vital component of outcome 5 for the advanced nurse practitioner (UKCC, 1994). As the advanced nurse practitioner is empowering staff to act in the best interests of clients, he or she is indirectly providing the authority to empower clients to take risks. It is essential therefore that the advanced nurse practitioner has a comprehensive knowledge of the strategies for assessing risks and that he or she is able to instruct and educate staff in the implementation of these strategies.

The advanced nurse practitioner – as a result of the power and autonomy that he or she possesses – is able to demonstrate impartiality when reviewing the benefits and risks to clients in potentially hazardous situations, and as a result is able to justify decisions made regarding risk-taking initiatives. This is a luxury that the RNMH often feels is lacking in their delivery of care, due partly to the direct, hands-on caring role and partly to the competing professional loyalties noted above. Once more, the concepts of empowerment and education of staff are seen to play a prominent role for the advanced nurse practitioner in ensuring safety and effectiveness of care provision and again the advanced nurse practitioner is in the position to influence the care of people with learning disabilities through the use of empowerment and education.

Table 17.1   Skills of the advanced nurse practitioner in learning disability nursing (Rich, 1996, adapted from UKCC, 1994).

Outcome 1: Set, implement and evaluate standards of nursing care across a range of care provision
Requires an ability to set and maintain high standards of care including:
- Comprehensive knowledge of a variety of quality assurance strategies
- Demonstrates ability in setting achievable, measurable standards of care and initiating quality assurance strategies
- Demonstrates proficiency in monitoring and auditing standards of care
- Demonstrates an ability to involve service-users, relatives, carers and professionals in setting and monitoring standards of care

Outcome 2: Lead the nursing team, where appropriate, to ensure effective management and professional development of the team and its resources
Requires an ability to identify a diversity of resources to assist in meeting client needs including:
- Comprehensive knowledge of a variety of resources to assist in meeting client needs
- Ability to co-ordinate resources to meet client needs
- Ability to prioritize use of resources as required
- Provides a comprehensive rationale for the use of resources

Outcome 3: Identify developmental need and potential and support and encourage primary and specialist practitioners to develop their practice
Requirements:
- Demonstrates clarity of vision and forward thinking in relation to operational and strategic planning
- Demonstrates an ability to develop and manage service level agreements for the provision of care
- Comprehensive knowledge of contracting and legal obligations of contracts
- Demonstrates an ability to motivate staff and gain commitment

Outcome 4: Initiate and lead practice developments to enhance safety and effectiveness in care and to identify individual and team development needs
Requires an ability to influence policy and decision-making
Requires comprehensive knowledge of a range of nursing models:
- Proficiently examines, analyses and evaluates a range of nursing models relevant to practices area
- Ability to compare and contrast various models of nursing
- Ability to relate models of nursing to other members of staff
Requires an ability to adapt and apply models of care to practice areas
- Proficiently applies models of nursing to practice
- Ability to adapt models of care to practice area
- Ability to evaluate the appropriateness of the model following application to practice area

Outcome 5: Supervise the clinical practice of the team to ensure safety and effectiveness in care and to identify individual and team development needs
Requires the ability to diffuse conflicts within the team and with other health care professionals and ability to carry out proficient and comprehensive risk assessments
- Comprehensive knowledge of strategies for assessing risks

Contd

Table 17.1   *Contd*

- Demonstrates impartiality when reviewing the benefits and risks to clients in potentially hazardous situations
- Ability to justify decisions made regarding risk-taking
- Comprehensive knowledge of the role of client advocate and conflicts within the nursing profession
- Possesses the authority to empower clients to take controlled risks
- Possess the authority to empower staff to take controlled risks on behalf of clients

Outcome 6: Manage the team to realise the full potential of individuals and the team as a whole
Requires proficient management/leadership skills
- Demonstrates ability to effectively manage change
- Demonstrates comprehensive problem-solving abilities
- Ability to liaise with other health care professionals in relation to operational and strategic planning
- Comprehensive knowledge of disciplinary procedures and an ability to effect procedures as necessary
- Demonstrates appropriate supervision and counselling of junior members of staff

Outcome 7: Identify, apply and disseminate research findings relating to clinical practice
Requires an ability to identify relevant research for practice area
- Comprehensive knowledge and understanding of recent nursing research appropriate to area of practice
- Ability to relate relevant research to others
- Ability to identify research areas required for area of practice
Requires an ability to apply relevant research to practice area
- Proficiently investigates, analyses and evaluates research appropriate to area of practice
- Proficiently applies and/or modifies relevant research to practice area
- Comprehensively documents the impact of research on care following application to practice area
- Proficiently carries out research within area of practice
- Comprehensive knowledge of ethical issues relating to implementing research studies and considers ethical implications prior to application of research to practice

Outcome 8: Ensure effective learning experience and environment for students of nursing
Requires an ability to plan and teach proficiently a range of education programmes
- Comprehensive knowledge of the principles of learning
- Proficiently prepares for practical and theoretical teaching sessions
- Provides a comprehensive range of resources for learners
- Demonstrates a comprehensive range of teaching strategies and methods
- Provides the required amount of support for learners according to stage of training
- Empowers learners to make justified moral decisions

Empowerment of staff, however, cannot occur without education, training, research and development. The UKCC (1994) highlight this in their standards for the advanced nurse practitioner (outcome 3) and stress that the individual must have an ability to:

'identify developmental need and potential and support and encourage primary and specialist practitioners to develop their practice.'

As an advanced nurse practitioner, therefore, it is necessary to demonstrate clarity of vision and forward thinking in relation to operational and strategic planning and to have an ability to encourage and motivate staff and gain staff commitment for future plans. In addition, the advanced nurse practitioner would be required to develop the practice of staff in order to fulfil their professional development and the developmental needs of the service.

The development of policies, procedures and philosophies of care should be based on best practice and research and, as noted above, should involve clinicians and care staff across the whole organization. The research and development role is emphasized in outcome 7 of the UKCC's standards for advanced nurse practitioners (UKCC, 1994). In practice, this is achieved by the possession of several key abilities:

(1)　A comprehensive knowledge and understanding of recent nursing research appropriate to the area of practice
(2)　An ability to disseminate relevant research to others
(3)　An ability to investigate, analyse and evaluate research appropriate to the area of practice
(4)　An ability to proficiently apply and/or modify relevant research to the practice area
(5)　An ability to identify research areas required for the area of practice
(6)　An ability to document the impact of research on care following the application to practice
(7)　An ability to proficiently carry out research within the area of practice
(8)　A comprehensive knowledge of ethical issues relating to implementing research studies

It must be emphasized, however, that research and development cannot be carried out in isolation, but must involve clinicians and care staff from the practice areas if staff are to feel committed to the unfolding philosophies of care and the policies and procedures of service provision.

The role of the advanced nurse practitioner in leading policy development is closely linked to quality assurance and outcome 1 of the UKCC's (1994) standards of the advanced nurse practitioner in which there is a requirement to:

'set, implement and evaluate standards of nursing care across a range of care provision'.

An advanced nurse practitioner needs to be involved in the setting, implementing and evaluating of standards of nursing care. This is particularly important within learning disabilities nursing owing to the diversity of disorders and disabling conditions encountered and, as a consequence, the diversity of care provision. As an advanced nurse practitioner, therefore, one must possess not only comprehensive knowledge of a variety of quality assurance strategies in order to set standards of care across such a wide range of care provision, but also an ability to involve service-users, relatives, carers and other professionals in setting and monitoring measurable and achievable standards of care.

The advanced nurse practitioner, therefore, influences direct care by being involved in the setting, implementation and evaluation of standards of nursing care, thus ensuring that the boundaries of care do not remain static and that current standards of care are moved forward to more adequately meet the needs of people with learning disabilities.

In addition to these skills, the advanced nurse practitioner must also demonstrate proficiency and impartiality in monitoring and evaluating standards of care in order to ensure a progressive movement of the boundaries of care provision. However, it must be stressed that the auditing of standards of care must also be carried out by an independent party to ensure an unbiased examination of standards.

It could be argued that there is an additional role for the advanced nurse practitioner in impartial freelance auditing of standards of care for other organizations, on the assumption that the advanced nurse practitioner is in an excellent position to evaluate standards of care. However, in practice this is not admissible due to the cut and thrust nature of the purchaser/provider climate of care provision for people with learning disabilities. The nature of this climate implies that if contracts are to be won, a good marketing strategy must be employed and a unique selling point (USP) emphasized. An advanced nurse practitioner can help promote and market the skills of professional and specialist nursing staff and can help to develop standards of care sufficiently to enable the service to become a flagship for future practice and potential leaders in the market of care, thus creating the required USP.

The management and leadership role of the advanced nurse practitioner is highlighted in outcomes 2 and 6 of the UKCC's standards (UKCC, 1994) which requires the advanced nurse practitioner to:

'lead the nursing team, where appropriate, to ensure effective management and professional development of the team and its resources' (outcome 2)

and to:

'manage the team to realise the full potential of individuals and the team as a whole' (outcome 6).

As an advanced nurse practitioner, this requires the ability to identify a diversity of resources to assist in meeting client needs and an ability to co-ordinate and prioritize the use of resources as required in addition to providing a comprehensive rationale for the use of these resources. In theory the authority to co-ordinate and prioritize the use of resources derives from the power-base and autonomy held by the advanced nurse practitioner; in practice, however, the provision of resources is dictated by the allocated budget.

One may assume that the advanced nurse practitioner requires proficient management skills in order to fulfil this role. However if, as noted above, the role of the advanced nurse practitioner is a joint lecturer-practitioner role with another organization (such as a university), management skills required are on the basis of consultancy or strategic management rather than hands-on operational management. Consultancy management nevertheless requires the advanced nurse practitioner to effectively initiate and manage change, particularly in developing policy and care philosophies, to have comprehensive problem-solving abilities, and to have an ability to liaise with other health care professionals.

In summary, the role of the advanced nurse practitioner in the field of learning disabilities can be described as (Rich, 1996):

- The key role of the advanced nurse practitioner is not necessarily that of a direct carer, but uses his or her position of power and authority to influence the care of people with learning disabilities through the use of empowerment and education.
- The advanced nurse practitioner possesses the ability, power, authority and autonomy to respond to both client and organizational needs, to develop and lead practice and to deal with morally difficult situations and ethical dilemmas.
- The advanced nurse practitioner is actively involved in the planning of service provision in order to ensure that contracts for care are won based on the highest possible standards of care, and not based on a low-cost factor which relies on less qualified but inexpensive staff.
- The advanced nurse practitioner is involved in marketing the skills and expertise available within the organization and ensures that where care has been improved through the application of research and development, the benefits to the clients and/or the organization have been highlighted and fully documented.
- The advanced nurse practitioner should also be involved in curriculum development and the teaching of courses leading to all levels of nursing practice (from professional level to advanced nurse practitioner level) to ensure that the content is appropriate to the field of learning disabilities.

References

Miller, B.K., Manson, T.J. & Lee, H. (1983) Patient advocacy – do nurses have the power and authority to act as patient advocates? *Nursing Leadership*, **6** (2).

Rich, F. (1996) The role of the advanced nurse practitioner in learning disability nursing. MSc dissertation. University of Central England, Birmingham.

UKCC (1994) *The Council's Standards for Education and Practice Following Registration.* Annex 1 to Registrar's letter 20/1994. UKCC, London.

Chapter 18

Advanced Practice in the Care of Older People

Patricia Elliott

Introduction

In 1992, amidst a background of the UKCC consultancy period regarding the PREP proposals (UKCC, 1993), I was appointed to the post of advanced nursing practitioner in the area of rehabilitation and care of older people, which for me resulted in the most fulfilling, stimulating and rewarding period in my 22 years of nursing. There was little empirical evidence or British literature as to the nature and value of the role. The American literature was therefore scanned in order to provide some insight as to how my role could develop. My hospital director gave me a free hand in taking forward nursing issues in order to improve patient services. The post initially was within the hospital but, ultimately, Trust wide. It was believed that if this role were successful in one hospital, it would provide a model to develop patient services in other areas of the Trust. At this time I was also pursuing a MSc degree, with an advanced nursing practice pathway which allowed me to critically analyse the role.

Defining the role

Although the concept of advanced nursing practice is complex, an attempt had to be made to define and clarify the role before it could be developed and its effectiveness evaluated. From the literature three main dimensions to the role clearly emerge. First, the way in which the sub-roles of clinical practice, education, nursing leadership and support, research, policy influencer and consultant are integrated to enhance patient care (Hamric & Spross, 1993; Menard, 1987).

The second dimension is the level of professional performance of the practitioner. There is an expectation that, with greater experience and knowledge, nurses will function at differing levels of skill. Table 18.1 attempts to identify functional levels within the period of preceptored

Table 18.1 Clinical practice levels.

Practice level	Education level	Cognitive level	Skill level	Experiential level
Preceptored practice	Diploma (2) Degree (3)	Knowledge Comprehension	Novice Professional Awareness	Exposure Participation
Professional practice	Diploma (2) Degree (3)	Application	Competent Professional Identity	Identification
Specialist practice	Degree (3) Masters (M)	Analysis Synthesis	Proficient Professional Maturity	Internalization
Advanced practice	Masters (M) PhD	Evaluation	Expert Professional Mastery	Dissemination

practice, professional practice, specialist practice and advanced practice (Bloom *et al.*, 1956; Benner, 1984; Sovie, 1983; Steinaker & Bell, 1979).

The third dimension is the scope and influence of the individual's practice. The advanced nursing practitioner should demonstrate 'best practice' within his or her own case-load, and also assist others to attain this goal (Bates, 1970). This can be achieved through consultation, paper writing and conference presentations. Having increased political and professional power can also positively influence nursing in a wider arena (Wallace & Gough, 1995).

These three dimensions provided a theoretical framework and foundation for the development of my new role as advanced nursing practitioner within a Community Trust. One exploratory study into the effectiveness of the role (Elliott, 1996) highlighted, in addition to these three dimensions of advanced nursing practice, that the personal qualities and attributes of the individual practitioner were also of significant importance. When attempting to motivate and empower others, it is essential to create a safe environment in which there is professional trust, a positive relationship and mutual professional respect. The role also demands flexibility and adaptability in order to respond to the ever-changing needs of patients, colleagues, the nursing profession and the society which a community hospital serves. The following two scenarios highlight how these three dimensions of advanced nursing practice were integrated to enhance nursing care within the hospital.

Scenario one: advancing resuscitation skills

While involved in my day to day clinical practice I became aware that many of the nurses were anxious regarding their responsibilities in the event of a cardiac arrest. Many of them had worked in the care of older people for a long time and had not experienced an arrest situation. Although arrests were not common they were becoming more frequent due to the changes in services provided at the hospital. A shambolic incident with one arrest situation confirmed that there was indeed justification for the anxiety.

Following the incident, I examined the protocols and policies regarding the cardiac arrest and found gaps and inaccuracies. New research-based guidelines were developed, following a search of the literature which reflected the United Kingdom resuscitation guidelines (Evans Medical, 1997), and staff were consulted and included throughout the whole process. The guidelines were presented at the Nursing Advisory Board for ratification.

Once the guidelines were ratified I was able to organize their launch and provide a series of educational workshops for all grades of staff. Regular simulation exercises (Megacode) were organized and these included all members who would normally be involved in the arrest scenario. A manikin was used allowing everyone to carry out their own role, just as they would in the real event. General practitioners who attended the hospital were involved in the Megacodes which helped update their own little used skills. It proved an excellent collaborative event. The simulation also provided a forum for nurses to discuss their anxieties and fears as well as develop and maintain essential skills.

The staff became so committed that money was raised to purchase a new defibrilatable manikin. Obtaining this manikin made the Megacodes even more realistic, allowing practice of all skills required in the arrest situation, defibrillation, intubation and cannulation in addition to CPR (cardiopulmonary resuscitation). I then began to audit the arrests within the hospital, the findings confirming that the management of the arrest situation in the hospital had improved 100%. This example of a clinical problem necessitated the integration of the sub-roles, a depth of knowledge and experience and has had a Trust-wide impact. The integration of the sub-roles is summarized in Table 18.2.

Scenario two: advancing assessment skills

During a period of clinical supervision with nurses on a general practitioner medical ward, nurses were highlighting grave concerns regarding their accountability in situations of conflict between nurses and doctors. Nursing in a community hospital incurs a greater professional responsi-

Table 18.2 Example of the advanced nursing practitioner sub-roles.

Sub-role	Example in practice
Practitioner	Through the involvement in clinical practice, identified deficits in CPR management and practitioner anxiety.
Policy influencer	Took forward inadequacies in CPR guidelines, met with staff to develop new guidelines, linked with managers and presented the guidelines at the Nursing Advisory Board.
Educator	Conducted training needs analysis, set up training sessions for all grades of staff followed up with Megacode sessions.
Researcher	Conducted literature search to gain an evidence base for practice. Conducted an arrest audit and skills audit.
Disseminator of information	Took new guidelines to meetings. Launched them through staff workshops.
Clinical supervisor	Through a process of one-to-one clinical supervision, assisted staff through the reflective process to identify a way to resolve their anxieties.
Professional leader	Took a clinical problem, arrived at a solution, motivated staff to purchase equipment. Implemented a system of nursing intervention which more adequately met the needs of the patient in the arrest situation. Gave nurses greater competence and confidence in the management of cardio-pulmonary resuscitation.
Flexibility	Through identifying priorities and being adaptable and flexible with the ability to straddle management education and practice, allowed resolution of the clinical problem.

bility as there is no resident doctor. It is therefore less easy to access medical advice than in a large acute hospital setting.

On investigation it was apparent that the doctors believed they were being inappropriately summoned to see patients in the ward, while the nurses quite rightly demanded medical attention for medical problems. There was an inconsistency in referrals, with the least experienced staff being perceived by the doctors as demanding a visit for trivial issues. During the course of working with this group of nurses, I observed that there were problems with attitudes of some doctors towards nurses. I also observed that some nurses, although they had an intuitive feel (Benner,

1984) that a patient's condition was changing, were inadequate at articulating this to the medical staff. On one occasion while working on the ward, I overheard the following telephone conversation as a nurse was requesting a doctor to visit:

'Sorry to bother you. Can you call in and see Mr Smith. I'm a bit worried about him, he's not very well today; he's just not right, he's very chesty.'

The medical staff, in order to make an informed decision regarding the priority of a visit against the conflicting demands on their time, required comprehensive information communicated in an appropriate language. This situation was a source of irritation to both doctors and nurses.

In an attempt to resolve some of the tensions, I drew on an observation I made when visiting the USA to explore the advanced practitioner role. The American baccalaureate and master's-prepared nurses were equipped to conduct full health assessments which included a physical examination, using the skills of inspection, palpation, auscultation and percussion. This is an area not included in British pre-registration preparation. The West Midlands Region in 1996 took a lead in introducing to the UK the concept of physical examination to Master's degree students.

Following discussions with the nurses it was felt that they would gain greater confidence in their decisions to seek medical help if these were supported by objective findings obtained through physical examination of the patient. They believed this would help them articulate more effectively the need for a visit and that the doctors would have objective evidence on which to base and prioritize their decisions.

I was then able, due to my educational background, to develop a pilot course aimed at providing registered nurses with physical examination skills. The course was successful and the nurses realized its potential in resolution of the recent problems. The course's success was demonstrated when I witnessed the following telephone conversation as one of the course participants rang a doctor:

'Mr Jones is complaining of pain on inspiration, and he has a sore throat; his pharynx is red, he has a temperature of 38.6, pulse 84 and respiration is 26. He has no cyanosis, but is breathless on slight exertion. He has normal breath sounds throughout both lung fields with occasional coarse crackles in the right upper lobe. Could you pop in and see him?'

The nurse was able to confidently communicate in an objective manner, giving the doctor information on which to base his decision to visit. This course has now been accredited and attracts 15 CAT (credit accumulation transfer) points at level 3. Through working on the ward with the nurses following the courses, I was able to supervise practice and help in determining the practical application of physical examination to everyday situations.

Helping nurses to develop physical examination skills aims to enhance nursing and is in no way taking over the medical role. Overall being able to make more detailed observations and being able to articulate findings more effectively should create a better working partnership between medical and nursing team members.

Despite the benefits of better communication and earlier identification of patient problems, there have been mixed responses from doctors to the nurses' newly-developed skills. Some have been extremely encouraging and supported nurses in supervising skills practice. Some have inappropriately expected nurses to take on roles that they were not confident to undertake. A small number have expressed concern at nurses undertaking what they perceive as a medical role which has taken doctors 5 years to perfect.

Attempts have been made to reassure medical staff that the skills nurses are now using are practised within a nursing framework and are not aimed at medical diagnosis and prescription. The nurse's aim is to identify states which deviate from normal health and to describe that state in an objective and professional manner, while also using the information to provide a comprehensive nursing care plan. The integration of the advanced practitioner sub-roles in this scenario is summarized in Table 18.3.

Conclusion

I hope I have been able to demonstrate through these two scenarios how I took the complex concept of advanced nursing practice to produce a workable definition to guide my role development. The aim of the role is to develop and advance nursing practice for the benefit of patients. It was through the integration of the sub-roles of practitioner, educator, professional leader, policy influencer and clinical supervisor that significant practice developments were facilitated.

The success of the post of advanced nursing practitioner in the community hospital has been seen by Trust managers and has been considered as a model for the rest of the Trust. In 1997 two further advanced nursing practitioners were appointed. It must be remembered as we develop the advanced nursing practitioner role that it must be driven by the genuine need to improve nursing care. In advancing nursing we must acknowledge the Code of Conduct (UKCC, 1992) by asking as we contemplate each new innovation, 'Is it in the best interest of the patient?' When seeking to expand and advance our role, especially as nurses take on roles previously regarded as medical, we must clearly focus on the essence of that special art and science of 'nursing'.

Table 18.3 An example of the integration of the advanced nursing practitioner sub-roles.

Sub-role	Example in practice
Practitioner	Involvement in practice, analytical ability, and knowledge and skill in physical examination assisted in identification of clinical need.
Policy influencer	Influence regarding clinical supervision for nurses and provision of a policy for E grade nurses to undertake physical examination training.
Educator	Development and organization of course, teaching on course, and negotiated module accreditation for CAT points.
Disseminator	Through teaching in the module and paper writing on the subject.
Researcher	Literature searching around the area of doctor/nurse relationships and nurses' skill levels. Auditing the effectiveness of the module.
Clinical supervisor	Provision of one-to-one clinical supervision with the aim of supporting and developing practitioners while also monitoring best practice.
Professional leader	Taking up problematic areas such as the conflicting demands between doctors and nurses, highlighting potential solutions and leading nurses into new areas of practice aimed at enhancing nursing care.

References

Bates, B. (1970) Doctors and nurses: changing roles and relations. *New England Journal of Medicine*, **283** (3), 129–34.

Benner, P. (1984) *From Novice to Expert Excellence and Power in Clinical Nursing Practice*. Addison Wesley, Menlo Park.

Bloom, B.S., Crathwohl, D.R. *et al.* (1956) *A Taxonomy of Educational Objectives, Handbook 1 and 2*. Longman, Harlow.

Elliott, P.A. (1996) *Celebrating success and cascading confidence: an exploratory study into the effectiveness of the advanced nursing practitioner role through clinical supervision*. Unpublished MSc dissertation, University of Central England in Birmingham.

Evans Medical (1997) *The RTO Resource File: A Guide to the 1997 Resuscitation Guidelines for Use in the United Kingdom*. Evans/IMS with the co-operation of the Resuscitation Council of the United Kingdom.

Hamric, A. & Spross, J. (eds) (1993) *The Clinical Nurse Specialist in Theory and Practice*. W.B. Saunders, Philadelphia.

Menard, S.W. (ed.) (1987) *The Clinical Nurse Specialist Perspectives on Practice*. John Wiley and Sons, New York.

Sovie, M. (1993) Professional development framework. *Journal of Nursing Staff Development,* **6**, 296–301.

Steinaker, N.W. & Bell, M.R. (1979) *The Experiential Taxonomy.* Academic Press, New York.

Wallace, M. & Gough, P. (1995) The UKCC criteria for specialist and advanced nursing practice. *British Journal of Nursing,* **16**.

UKCC (1992) *The Code of Professional Conduct.* United Kingdom Central Council for Nurses, Midwives and Health Visitors, London.

UKCC (1993) *The Scope of Professional Practice.* United Kingdom Central Council for Nurses, Midwives and Health Visitors, London.

UKCC (1994) *Post Registration Education and Practice.* United Kingdom Central Council for Nurses, Midwives and Health Visitors, London.

UKCC (1996) *PREP. The Nature of Advanced Practice, an Interim Report,* Colloquium 1, annex 4. United Kingdom Central Council for Nurses, Midwives and Health Visitors, London.

Chapter 19
Advanced Nursing Practice in A&E – How it Differs from Specialist and Professional Practice

Patricia Overton-Brown

Introduction

At the outset of the initial educational programme which was set to prepare me as an advanced nurse practitioner (ANP), I must confess my understanding of the concept was naive and elementary. I feel this is important as my limited understanding was attributable to the term 'advanced practice'. At that time this term suggested to me that the role of the ANP would be entirely rooted in the 'doing' of clinical practice. As the dawning appeared, which was a painful and uncomfortable educational process, I matured and evolved. On reflection, I do feel that the educational process prepared and offered me the opportunity to gain a greater knowledge and understanding of current issues affecting my area of clinical practice through the dimensions of advanced nursing.

This chapter is a personal account of my post-education developing role as an advanced nurse practitioner within an accident and emergency setting. I hope the sharing of part of my first six months of practice will reflect and demonstrate the kaleidoscopic nature of advanced practice, which is fluid, shifting and changing and can never be otherwise, and is not found in a fixed rigid definition of a title. I also hope to illustrate from my observations and experience my own perceptions of the distinguishing features of professional, specialist and advanced practice within A&E (Accident and Emergency) nursing.

Initially it was proposed within the A&E directorate, and also echoed from the nursing voice within the wider Trust, that my focus should be within the research dimension of advanced practice. As a clinical leader I possess a degree of research credibility, gained through the formalized educational system which prepared me for the role. My key objective was to pursue nursing development unit (NDU) status to advance professional practice within the A&E department through evaluation of practice, research and dissemination.

In an NDU, development of the nursing workforce is viewed as a vital component in working towards advancements in patient care. The supposition is that progress in the care setting is simultaneous with the development of the workforce. It was clear to me, as the clinical leader of the project, that the department needed to establish firm foundations to support a successful launch of such an initiative. Included among other preparatory work, it was necessary to ensure that appropriate education and teaching programmes were in place for staff development within the A&E department. My focus was then diverted to the teaching and educational dimension of advanced practice. This is the area where I have currently made most progress.

The education role in advanced practice

In the first instance, I explored the existing teaching arrangements and facilitated another team member in formulating a system where current in-house training initiatives could be formally documented and evaluated. I proceeded to undertake an educational audit and staff training development review. This allowed me to ascertain the current level of skills and knowledge within the unit. As an integral part of this process, I also elicited the nursing staffs' perceptions of their immediate training and educational requirements. I felt this was important in order to identify key result areas for professional development of clinical practice, highlighted by the practitioners themselves. This was an interesting and enlightening exercise and supplied me with a wealth of information. Using this information I proposed a departmental policy for consultation which offered a structured framework for development of nursing staff of all grades. Such an initiative, if accepted and resourced, also has the potential to retain a highly trained/skilled workforce in a competitive market.

I envisage that this structured framework will cover the range from novice professional practitioner through to the development of the specialist practitioner. This will offer a more organized approach to skills training, teaching and education within the A&E unit. Currently I have introduced a two week intensive induction programme for new D grade staff nurses. Table 19.1 shows the content of the induction programme.

This programme is designed to complement the existing preceptor/ mentorship induction arrangements. In support of this initiative, many experienced staff have contributed to the content and delivery. In addition, a culture change is now evident in the understanding, through my facilitation of declaration of competencies within expanded role functions. This is now more fully understood by all staff, and certainly by the new practitioners, as no longer one of assessment and certification of the practitioner by the medical profession, but one of autonomous practice and the pro-

Table 19.1 Content of induction programme.

Day 1	Introduction to A&E Tour of the unit/hospital Roles and relationships Fears and expectations
Day 2	Revisit fears and expectations Principles of A&E nursing Triage Walking wounded Policies and procedures departmental/hospital
Day 3	Bone healing and fracture management Plastering techniques Wound care and management Suture workshop
Day 4	Scope of Professional Practice Ethical and legal issues for nurses in A&E The role of the nurse in the resus. room Observations The nurse's role in the initial assessment of major trauma scenarios
Day 5	Basic airway maintenance Basic life support The nurse and the interpretation of ECGs Feedback and reflective practice Evaluation and overview of the week
Day 6	Mentorship and induction First clinical placement The role of the nurse in dealing with paediatrics in A&E The Childrens Act
Day 7	The role of the nurse in dealing with the shocked patient Head injuries Scavenger hunt Dealing with deliberate self harm Dealing with aggression
Day 8	A&E nursing in the organization Second clinical placement The wider issues within the NHS Quality standards The nursing strategy
Day 9	The department strategy Role dimensions Ethical and legal issues Sudden death
Day 10	Stress in the workplace Assertiveness Third clinical placement Feedback and reflective practice

fessional accountability of the nurse. Examples of expanded role functions are shown in Table 19.2.

This for me has been a major breakthrough in advancing professional practice within the unit. I believe that *The Scope of Professional Practice* (UKCC, 1992a) and the revised *Code of Professional Conduct* (1992b) are little understood by the profession which has failed to realise that these documents removed the previous extended role straitjacket which surrounded developments in professional nursing practice.

Table 19.2   Expanded role functions.

Plastering	Suturing
Cannulation	Blood letting
Intravenous drug administration	Defibrillation
Referral to other health care agencies	Requesting radiographs
Administration of medicines within agreed protocols	Clinical assessment and management of minor extremity trauma

My links with the local university are strong and I played a key role in the curriculum planning and validation committee of the post-registration accident and emergency course. This gave me the opportunity to influence the indicative content of the course to ensure that it met service requirements. Contractual agreements have ensured that this course now plays a key link in the ongoing education and clinical career development of A&E staff, incorporated within my overall vision of a structured framework towards specialist practice.

Developments in accident and emergency nursing

The emergency nurse practitioner (ENP) is a trained experienced nurse who assesses, treats and discharges certain types of patients attending A&E, without referring them to a doctor. The department has an in-house ENP module of study also academically accredited by the university. I have been involved in the delivery of that module and also developed a tool to evaluate the training as well as the clinical supervision and assessment strategy in place. For the future, I foresee the evolution of this module, perhaps within the university setting to ensure more accessibility for A&E nurses. This could be developed and incorporated into an honours degree programme of study which could fully embrace the concept of specialist practitioner in A&E.

To support my 'structured framework' for education and development within the clinical setting, I firmly believe in the need for clinical supervision. The concept, of course, like many other issues related to professional practice, requires careful planning. To date I have been involved in project pilot work in the main developing, monitoring and evaluation systems, to introduce clinical supervision in my employing Trust. A&E will be one of eight pilot sites for this initiative.

Within A&E circles there has recently been a move towards the establishment of a national triage scale to standardize clinical priority of patients attending A&E departments. Having undertaken instructors' training with two other colleagues, I am now preparing to train the trainers within the department. As an ANP I foresee that I will be involved not only in the project planning and dissemination, but also in the evaluation of the new triage system, which I feel will become a requirement from the purchasers in the not too distant future.

In relation to the nursing care of the multiple traumatized patient, I am exploring the potential to hold a multi-disciplinary advanced trauma life support and advanced trauma nursing course within the Trust. This multi disciplinary approach to the treatment, management and care of the traumatized patient is a philosophy to which I am committed and I hope to use my instructor status to continue to disseminate and influence good practice locally and nationally.

Advanced v. specialist nursing practice in A&E

It is within the area of the 'doing' of advanced clinical practice that I have made least impact at present. The reasons for this are multi faceted. Indirectly, however, I feel I am working towards improving the efficiency and effectiveness of practice for the benefit of patients through the dimensions of advanced practice in teaching and education. Although I have concentrated on one dimension of practice to give the reader a flavour of the evolution of the role of the ANP, Figure 19.1 illustrates how inter-related the dimensions of practice are, and the concept has to be appreciated as part of the whole.

It might be argued that all practising nurses have a responsibility to help others within the profession to learn, and indeed, teaching is an integral part of nursing. Asked then to differentiate this aspect in relation to professional, specialist and advanced practice, I believe I can offer a personal viewpoint to stimulate further discussion based on observation of professional practice and personal experience.

A&E nursing is diverse. Patients present with a wide range of conditions which vary from those requiring life-saving interventions to basic first-aid. It has been my observation that the professional nurse entering the A&E setting requires a lengthy period to develop confidence in the practical skills and knowledge needed to care for such patients. It is only once

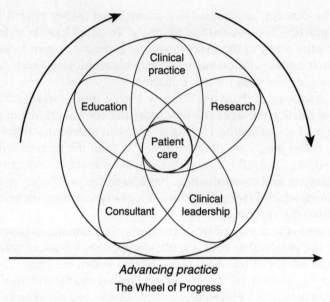

Advancing practice
The Wheel of Progress

Fig. 19.1   Interrelated dimensions of advanced practice.

expertise is gained from experience that the professional nurse begins to share it, usually through mentorship and preceptorship. In my experience, this teaching and sharing of knowledge is rarely evident until a recognized course in teaching and assessing has been completed. The professional nurse in A&E does teach and educate, but from a basis of their experiences within the department.

In relation to specialist practice, I have the following observations to offer. Many patients attend A&E with illness or injury and are seeking treatment or cure. Much of the work therefore has a medical model focus. Clinical nursing expertise and teaching is evident within the areas of resuscitation, trauma nursing, cardiac specialism and ENPs in the treatment of minor extremity trauma. Many of these experts would consider themselves clinical specialists, defining their specialist role by the performance of clinical practice rather than from the knowledge base from which they act. While many have undertaken educational programmes to support this knowledge base and experience, the focus remains reductive in its approach and does not fully embrace the nursing framework for specialist practice laid out by the higher award.

I believe this is important if, as a profession, we are to avoid the development of nursing roles that are recognized as specialists with a purely pathophysiological orientation. In summary, some clinical nurse specialists demonstrate evidence of fulfilling the standards for specialist practice; however, many more do not. Are these nurses specialists in a specialist area or professional nurses working within a specialist area?

My appreciation of advanced practice is of a more 'holistic' or 'global' approach to advancing professional nursing practice towards improvements in patient care, based on all of the dimensions:

- Clinical practice
- Clinical education
- Clinical research
- Clinical consultancy
- Clinical leadership

This I feel will be determined in the future by research and evaluation. ANPs perceive the development of nursing through their conceptualization of nursing and the profession's values and philosophy. Perhaps the difference can be attributed to the ideology and vision which drives the individual. That individual too needs to be articulate and skilled in debate, and knowledgeable of the political and policy making arenas to move the profession forward. I belive this is the role of the ANP.

In summary, I feel as a profession we need to be careful not to create boundaries. The future of professional practice is dependent on all professionals, specialists and advanced nurse practitioners working in collaboration, to complement and not compete, in order to meet the needs of our society. In a health service driven by competition, cost containment and quality assurance, surrounded by legal and ethical debate as well as increasing revolutionary technology, the profession has many barriers to overcome without instituting intraprofessional rivalry.

Part 4
The Future

Chapter 20
The Future of Specialist and Advanced Practice

George Castledine

Introduction

Increasing specialization was justified in medicine because doctors felt they could not become good enough at all the different things they had to do. In some ways this is also true in nursing, as some nurses have developed specialist roles in response to the medical division of labour. Others, such as the cancer care nurse, may be products of a specialization that follows from a condition needing on-going nursing management as the patient goes through a number of treatments.

There is a danger that some nurse specialists focus their work too much on the medical model and the technical medical procedures associated with that approach. On the other hand, there are those who maintain very much a nursing perspective and emphasize the application of a higher level of nursing competence. Something very serious is happening to core nursing tasks. This is partly the result of increased patient turnover, the shortage of qualified nurses and the present system of nurse training, and partly because nurses are being constantly encouraged to take on more medical tasks. Whatever the reasons, nurse specialists of the future should be acting as clinical leaders, promoting the development and application of the essentials of nursing.

Developing the role

It is important for specialist and advanced nurses to remember that nursing is about nurturing and helping patients. These aspects of nursing practice must be integrated into the new developments in nursing's knowledge and skill. It is essential that nurses are dynamic and assertive in their total nursing care role and that they do not become the technical substitutes of physicians.

The International Council of Nurses (ICN, 1992) published a list of the forces driving the creation of nursing specialties, dividing them into two – those forces external to nursing and those within the profession (Table 20.1).

The United Kingdom Central Council specialist working group (UKCC, 1997) carried out an extensive consultation exercise and found that there was strong consistency and consensus around the following key issues with regard to the present and future direction of specialist nurses in the UK:

(1) There was a lack of a common understanding or agreement regarding the role, responsibilities or preparation of nurse practitioners and clinical nurse specialists. There also appeared to be no common job descriptions for either remit, even within individual trusts. While several people held firm views as to what they considered the roles were about, their views did not necessarily concur.

(2) The considerable confusion around the present UKCC arrangement for specialist practice, including transitional arrangement, with widely differing interpretation of the implementation of the standards.

(3) The need for clarity by employers as well as the profession as to whether specialist practice relates to levels, roles or responsibilities.

(4) The difficulties around the title of specialist practice and its resulting association and thus confusion with specialism, specialty and specialist.

Table 20.1   Forces driving the creation of nursing specialties.

External to nursing	Professional
Increased complexity of health care	Development of nursing science and knowledge/research
Changing health needs, e.g. new diseases, demographic changes	Extension of boundaries of nursing practice, e.g. primary health care
Health policy decisions, e.g. focus on primary health care services	Development of post-basic curricula
Structural changes in health care system, e.g. development of trauma, dialysis, transplant centres	Search for improved career progression
New technologies	Search for more recognition by obtaining better:
Delegation by medical profession	• financial reward
Advances of medical practice and creation of new medical specialties	• authority and status
Availability of funds	Servicing and/or paralleling medical specialties
Consumer demand	Affiliation movements
Political interests, e.g. responses to lobbying by interest groups	
Product merchandizing	

(5) The potential negative effect on public confidence caused by the current confusion.
(6) A need to give due recognition to clinical practice within specialist practice as it is practice centred.
(7) Based on the above, the necessity to develop:
   - appropriate assessment strategies for practice to enable recognition of clinical practice
   - an end award that is practice-led with underpinning supportive education.

The UKCC also found that even since their published standards on post registration (UKCC, 1994), several other factors had come into consideration. For example, there had been an escalation and proliferation of specialist roles undertaken by nurses. Doctors were now beginning to share more of their work with nurses and the rest of the health care team, resulting in a blurring of traditional professional boundaries.

The UKCC's *Scope of Professional Practice* document (UKCC, 1992) is also having a positive effect in encouraging all nurses to develop their roles. This has led many people to believe that the UKCC should not be setting future guidelines which may hamper and restrict what is seen as a very flexible and enabling situation.

The nature of professional education for nurses has also changed substantially in the UK. There is now a definite drive towards an all-graduate profession with at least the majority of nurse specialists in the future holding a first degree. Nurses seem hungry for knowledge and qualifications, but we have to be careful that possession of a qualification or the completion of a course is not seen as the only criteria for the recognition of a specialist nurse.

The UKCC (1997), in the recommendations of their report, emphasize the importance of clearly articulating what is meant by specialist and advanced practice. They certainly feel that what the profession and other interested stakeholders are referring to is a 'level of practice'. This point was supported by the review team who were commissioned by the four health departments in the UK to conduct a review of the Nurses, Midwives and Health Visitors Act:

'We recognize that this is a difficult area which the profession will have to debate for itself. Our view, as outsiders to the profession, is that it could make sense to define one or two additional levels of professional competence (but not more) perhaps recognizing the two aspects of the senior or advanced practitioner who has developed his or her competencies well beyond the minimum level acquired at the point of registration.' (J.M. Consulting Ltd, 1998)

Work is urgently needed to identify the competencies of specialist and advanced practice. Literature in this area is scarce, although there have been attempts by Fenton (1985) and Klein (1994), for example, using Benner's (1984) areas of skilled performance which reflect expert practice based on the Dreyfus model of skill acquisition.

Specialization in health care has traditionally been associated with the development of the hospital. It was in the German speaking countries in the mid 1880s, such as in Vienna, where specialism in medicine was pioneered coupled with a rigorous scientific approach based in hospitals, which became the scientific laboratories for doctors (Konner, 1993).

The effectiveness of specialized hospital medicine grew when nursing became a hospital-based profession, and it helped to establish the scientific basis of sterile technique and infection control. Some specialists, including surgeons, anaesthetists, radiologists and clinical pathologists, became so inseparable from their hospitals that many hospitals' reputations were made on the backs of the medical staff who worked in them. The obsession with hospitalized health care continued and strengthened even more when medical and nursing training was based in them.

Only over the last 10 years or so has hospital dominated care really been questioned as the most appropriate way to run a health service. Escalating costs have forced the government in the UK to reappraise the role and future of the hospital in the National Health Service. Many hospitals were considered out of date and inappropriate for the new style of hospital care in the next century. Long term care facilities were closed and the care of the chronically ill and infirm was transferred into the independent sector with the evolution of the nursing home and hospice. The trend in some countries, such as in North America, towards specialization and sub-specialization based on hospitals and away from primary care in the community, is causing major concerns and difficulties for a change of direction. In many rural and inner city areas in the USA there is a shortage of general practitioners, a fact which is also starting to occur in the UK.

The Government White Paper (1997) on the future of the NHS emphasizes the important new role of primary care, and the shift in emphasis away from hospitals:

'By empowering local doctors, nurses and health authorities to plan services we will ensure that the local NHS is built around the needs of patients. Hospitals and other agencies providing services will have a hand in shaping these plans but their primary duty will be to meet patients' requirements for high quality and easily accessible services. The needs of patients not the needs of institutions will be at the heart of the new NHS.'

With the development of new primary care groups, which will link with social services and NHS Trusts, there will be even greater opportunities for specialist nurses in the community. Nursing is at a critical stage in its development. It now has to grasp the opportunities which are rapidly becoming available. There is a need for traditional nurse specialists in the community, such as the health visitor and school nurse, to become much more flexible and proactive in the way they work. In hospital too, just working in a particular specialist field does not make a nurse a clinical expert:

'There is a clear difference between practising within a speciality and being a nursing specialist.' (UKCC, 1994)

The type of specialist nurse which bodies like the UKCC envisage is someone working at a different level, either in the community or in a hospital. It is probably inappropriate and confusing to call such a nurse a 'specialist' because so many other nurses are now using this title. What is needed is a more bland title, such as 'senior clinical nurse', for someone who has at least 5 to 10 years' clinical experience, has achieved a reasonable academic level, is respected and consulted by their colleagues and fits the criteria as laid out by the UKCC. Such an individual will certainly exercise a high level of judgement, discretion and decision-making in clinical care. They will be able to monitor and improve standards of nursing in various ways, such as audit and clinical supervision. Furthermore, they will be the clinical leaders of nursing care and the prime movers in developing practice, through research, teaching and the support of professional colleagues. Some of these senior clinical nurses will use skills and practices previously the domain of medicine. This does not make them into mini doctors but gives them an opportunity to provide a unique blend and broader scope of holistic health care.

The practice of senior clinical nurses in the future will cut across traditional nursing boundaries, ranging from forming closer relationships with physicians in clinics and private practices, to working with schools and staff in nursing homes and various other social and community services. The central theme of their practice will be total health care and wellness. Even in very specialized hospital services the senior clinical nurse will be the team leader and developer who not only is an expert in their field, but also acts like a consultant in nursing to colleagues across the health care disciplines, linking with management.

There will be some nurses who inevitably will align themselves with medicine and lose their identity as nurses. There is a place for such individuals within the health service as paramedical nurses, doctor's assistants or medical technicians. This minority should not be allowed to detract from the excellent work which the recognized senior clinical nurses will be doing. By incorporating a medical and nursing approach to care, senior clinical nurses are liberating themselves and becoming truly autonomous. On the other hand, if the nurses move too much towards a medical model dominating their care, they will become supervisors and will be governed by medicine.

Framework for a clinical career structure

A three-band clinical career structure for nursing could be the way forward. Within each band there should be the opportunity for nurses not only to move around without financial penalty, but also to gain wide experience and take on key leadership and clinical management tasks. Fig. 20.1 is a diagrammatic representation of this proposal.

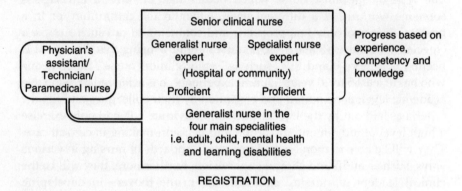

Fig. 20.1 Framework for a clinical career structure. (The senior clinical nurse (upper box) works at a higher level of practice; generalist and specialist nurses (lower two boxes) work at a standard or core level of nursing practice.)

Such a structure should allow nurses to develop their knowledge and competence and give them an opportunity to specialize in a particular field of nursing or area of practice. Some nurses may want to stay in a broader, generalist area of nursing and yet still develop their level of knowledge and competence. Fig. 20.1 demonstrates how this can be achieved.

When nurses register they enter one of four specialist areas – adult, child, mental health and learning disabilities – as a generalist practitioner. Some nurses will only want to achieve competence at this first generalist stage in their careers. This is totally acceptable, as long as they meet the requirements of PREP and keep up to date and maintain their standards as a first-stage generalist.

However, nurses who want to pursue their careers further can move into the second stage of practice by either continuing on their generalist profile or moving into a specialist nursing practice area. Whichever area they move into, they must improve their level of knowledge and competence. In future, this will usually be accomplished under the terms of PREP by taking a course at first-degree level that is recognized by the national boards.

Specialist and generalist nurses should also be allowed to move from one specialist area of practice to another. With the help of their profile, they should be able to demonstrate the relevant transferable skills and development of higher levels of competency and knowledge.

Progression through specialization or generalization at this stage should be based not only on continuing education and development but also on application to practice and experience. If the present clinical grading system was abolished, a more dynamic interpersonal and individual performance review system could be introduced. The key areas for role development into advanced nursing practice are clinical expertise, education, research, leadership, management and consultation.

The different types of specialist practitioner in the future will vary according to the public's demand for nursing. There is already a growing concern and reaction to the current disease-oriented, physician-controlled system. People are demanding more information and involvement in their local health care system. There is a need to stop the fragmentation of nursing into a vast number of different specialists. The future will see a much more dynamic multiskilled professional nurse who is able to work across previous nursing boundaries. She or he will be educated alongside other health and social care workers including doctors. While collaborative interprofessional services will flourish there will be the possibility for the development of senior clinical nurses working in independent nursing practices.

Perhaps Schlotfeldt's (1973) definition of nursing best sums up the future focus of the nurses' practice possibility into the next millennium:

'The nurses' practice focus should be on assessing people's health status, assets and deviations from health and on helping sick people to regain health and the will or near will to maintain or attain health through the selective application of nursing science and the use of available nursing strategies.'

There is a desperate need for senior clinical nurses to be taking the lead in caring for those patients who are suffering the long term effects of chronic disease. Nursing interventions should therefore be directed at the situations and problems that result from these disease processes and not just the medical treatments associated with the diagnostic label. Inherent in this approach is a need for future nurses to be more family orientated in their assessment and nursing care. Assessment and intervention in the local community and the patient's home provides an exciting opportunity for influencing local health care policy and neighbourhood sensitivity. More senior clinical nurses working closely alongside senior social workers may seem like an unrealistic aim at present, but it is a crucial outcome to work towards.

Nurses have a unique and special caring perspective of the patient, and their family and friends. It is an appropriate time for the specialists of the future to grasp the opportunities that are available and lead nursing into the twenty-first century.

References

Benner, P. (1984) *From Novice to Expert*. Addison-Wesley, Menlo Park.

Fenton, M.V. (1985) Identifying competencies of clinical nurse specialists. *Journal of Nursing Administration*, **15** (12), 31–7.

ICN (1992) *Guidelines on Specialisation in Nursing*. International Council of Nurses, Geneva.

J.M. Consulting Ltd (1998) *The Regulation of Nurses, Midwives and Health Visitors*, para 6, 10. J.M. Consulting Ltd, Bristol.

Klein, D.G. (1994) Critical care clinical nurse specialist: novice to expert. In: *The Clinical Nurse Specialist in Critical Care* (eds A. Garlinski & L.S. Kern). W.B. Saunders, Philadelphia.

Konner, M. (1993) *The Trouble with Medicine*. BBC Books, London.

Scholtfeldt, R.M. (1973) Planning for progress. *Nursing Outlook*, **21**, 766–9.

UKCC (1992) *The Scope of Professional Practice*. UKCC, London.

UKCC (1994) *The Future of Professional Practice*. The Council's standards for education and practice following registration. UKCC, London.

UKCC (1997) *PREP – Specialist Practice*. Considerations of issues relating to embracing nurse practitioners and clinical nurse specialists within the specialist practice framework. CC/97/46. UKCC, London.

White Paper (1997) *The New NHS, Modern, Dependable*. HMSO, London.

Index